Praise for *Don't Just Sit There, DO NOTHING*

"*Don't Just Sit There, DO NOTHING* covers the gamut of human emotion—Jessie writes so honestly about experiences that all of us can relate to. Plus, she delves into the ancient wisdom of the Tao Te Ching that shows us how to let go of resentments, of the past, of the 'what-ifs' and the 'should'ves.' She takes us through her painful, hilarious, miraculous journey, shining light on our own. She shares the epiphanies that have changed her life and that can change ours, too. She pieces together fun and humor (celebrity run-ins, Hollywood sets) with darker subjects (her immigration, eating disorder, date rape) much like life itself does. Get ready for a ride!"

—Karen Salmansohn, multibestselling author
and award-winning designer

"Jessie Kanzer's refreshing voice carries a clarity and candidness that pulls you in—that makes room for the unseen magic in life as it unfolds."

—Erin Khar, managing editor at Ravishly

"Jessie Kanzer's book, as well as her personal story, are inspiring, insightful and beautifully written. For anyone looking to connect more to their higher self, I highly recommend reading this!"

—Serena Dyer Pisoni, author of *The Knowing* and
Don't Die with Your Music Still in You

"Jessie Kanzer shares funny, frank, and engaging stories of her exile from the Soviet Union, finding spirituality, serenity, and love as an American wife and mom."

—Susan Shapiro, bestselling author of *Unhooked* and
The Forgiveness Tour

Don't Just Sit There, DO NOTHING

Don't Just Sit There,

DO NOTHING

Healing, Chilling & Living
with the Tao Te Ching

JESSIE ASYA KANZER

Foreword by Laura Day

HAMPTON ROADS

Cover and text design by Kathryn Sky-Peck
Typeset in Adobe Text Pro

Hampton Roads Publishing Company, Inc.
Charlottesville, VA 22906
Distributed by Red Wheel/Weiser, LLC
www.redwheelweiser.com

ISBN: 978-1-64297-035-7
Library of Congress Cataloging-in-Publication Data available upon request.

Printed in the United States of America
IBI
10 9 8 7 6 5 4 3 2 1

For Gigi, Charlie, and Adam (and our cat Regis—Charlie made me add him even though I told her he'll never be able to read) . . . and for Mama, Papa, Sasha, and Babushka.

That is the bread of the Jessie Asya sandwich.

Contents

IDENTITY

AWARENESS

CREATION

Foreword

I do not write forewords. I am pathologically exacting, and I seldom agree with enough of the book—or enough of its author—to feel comfortable setting my recommendation in indelible ink.

But when Jessie asked me to write this foreword, I was overcome by an intuitive feeling. A "yes" escaped my lips before I had time to think about it. I had not read a single line, yet I somehow knew that I would be struck by her book's honesty, clarity, and usefulness.

I was.

Jessie herself will not know, until she reads this foreword, that I remember her from long ago.

She would pop up at unexpected times in my groups and presentations, or by email. These were unremarkable sightings. Many of my students make sure I'm aware when they're around. Jessie was not one of them.

The Circle, my community, provides many open spaces for newcomers, especially for the young. It welcomes and embraces them. But Jessie was not immediately embraced. She was not outwardly needy. The tidy way she hid her pain, expressing it in well-crafted sentences instead of colorful drama, was not directly inviting. Quietly, though, she held her place, offered what she had to give, and learned from every turned back until she had accumulated a gift so great that the others had no choice but to turn around and see her.

This book is that gift. This honest, magnificent journey of courage and insight. The unveiling of light in a way that illuminates the light in each of us.

Jessie's message is simple. Good is searching for you. Let it in. Good is in you. Let it out.

Don't Just Sit There. Do Nothing.

Sometimes striving, doing, becomes a lack-of-faith vote against your own potential and against us, the ones who share this journey with you.

Jessie's writing style carries the reader effortlessly to a new way of being. Her prose eases and delights. "Some woman ran a red light and smashed her wheels straight into the middle of my ennui," she remarks of a traumatic accident that changed her life.

Children love heroes because they offer the hope of salvation and affirm our worthiness to be saved. In the end, our heroes are rarely the adrenaline-fueled people who jump into rushing waters to save our puppy, but rather the people who offer a moment of kindness, a leg up, or an example of resilience. The tenacity, day by day, to address quotidian challenges that seem to take us nowhere and give us nothing requires a truly intrepid soul. Courage is the ability to hope when we have been defiled and to move forward when there is no dream in sight. Courage is the determination to give what you have, even if it is found wanting, and to continue to improve it and offer it until it becomes the seed of someone else's hope.

I think you will find a hero in this book. And that hero is you.

—Laura Day
August 1, 2021
Sitting here. Doing nothing. Joining you in same.

Introduction

One of the many idiosyncrasies of my life is that I was born without religion. I mean, I'm Jewish ethnically and traditionally—and I definitely feel my ancestral Jewishness. But in the Soviet Union, where I come from, that meant little else than a kick-in-the-butt of anti-Semitism. The fact is, I hail from a weird experiment of a society where religion was not allowed. Obviously the "not allowed" part is not ideal. But because God was never discussed (Lenin was) nothing was ever attributed to a power greater than myself. By the time I left that land to come to America, no amount of Hebrew School or Christmas carols, for that matter, could make me believe in a bearded man in the sky. In this way I was lucky. I was a blank slate.

Still, as I faced challenges, I wanted explanations. Like many of us, I longed for absolutes. In my search, I fell flat on my face more times than I care to recall—except, I recall them all in this book. It was at my lowest point, face down on the bathroom tiles, that I discovered the ancient teachings of the Tao Te Ching—enigmatic verses that gently shifted me in the right direction, which sometimes was no direction at all. Today, they continue to show me the value of *not* knowing, of simply existing and trusting. They encourage us all to go with the flow of life itself, so that we can move beyond the expectations and limitations we've grown so accustomed to. It's not that we stop working, it's that the work gets easier. Life gets easier.

Here, I've chosen some of my favorite verses of the Tao Te Ching, The Book of the Way, to help anchor us in the magic of this Tao, this *Way*, as it pertains to modern existence. I looked through dozens of translations of this second most translated text in the world (after the Bible) and decided to present its teachings through the lens of one girl's experience. The girl is me, the stories are mine, but the struggle is universal.

If you want to dive deeper into the Tao itself, take a look at the Acknowledgments section for titles of both well-known and obscure translations that helped me along. Though if I had to choose just one, I'd go with the first translation I ever read: *Tao Te Ching, A New English Version* by Stephen Mitchell. (The pocket-sized edition is one of my favorite things ever!)

To me, The Book of the Way, which dates back to 6th century BC China, is a living philosophy—one that continues to be relevant as long as we continue to look at it, interpret it, analyze it in order to help us create more peace within and without. That was its purpose all along, I think—to start a neverending discussion.

There is only sparse information about its author Lao Tzu, which means "The Old Guy" (his actual name is unknown). Some modern scholars see him as a mythical figure who's likely the compilation of several people. In religious Taoism, he is viewed as a supreme deity. Either way, he—or they—left behind a deep yet simple guide for living. I call it the world's oldest self-help book.

"'He who talks doesn't know, he who knows doesn't talk'—that is what Lao Tzu told us in a book of five thousand words," said the poet and comedian, Hence Po Chu-i. "If he was the one who knew, how could he have been such a blabbermouth?"

Well, my book is ten times as wordy, so I am ten times the blabbermouth. Trust me, I am. All these words, however, only serve as pointers. They direct you to a natural way that you, yourself, can choose to walk—or not.

I spread my life out under a microscope here to vividly demonstrate the very Way that The Book of the Way refers to. In hindsight, it's plain to see where I veered off and what I learned in so doing. In hindsight, I fall in love with every pitfall. And I adore the stories of my life as dearly as I do existence itself. In studying my past, in chuckling at it, I am able to let it go, to release it, and to finally be whole, to be free, to be me.

I hope you can recognize yourself in this "me" or clearly see your own life lessons after reading this book. And I hope that you too will fall more in love with your imperfect path and your imperfect self, learning to shed all of it from time to time. Most of all—and in the most loving way possible—I hope these teachings will assist you in chilling the fuck out! At least, just a little bit. And then a little bit more, until you flow like the text suggests. And as your life continues to unfold, the Tao, or the Way, will speak for itself.

IDENTITY

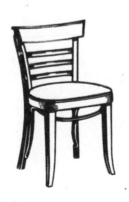

1

Gobbledygook

Ways that can be told are not the eternal Way.
Names that can be named must change with time and place.

The Nameless is the origin of Heaven and Earth.
Naming is the origin of all particular things.

Ever desireless, one can see the mystery.
Caught in desire, one sees only the manifestations.

Yet mystery and manifestations come from the same source;
though they bear different names, they serve the same
  mystical cause.

Mystery within mystery,
the gateway to all understanding.

—TAO TE CHING, VERSE 1

Or, as this immigrant knows (two thumbs pointing at my silly, insecure self):

The name that others can pronounce is not the real name. Labels may cover up the mystery, but it's still there, waiting to be unearthed.

Embracing the Mystery

"Gobbledygook," my husband Adam balks when I begin reading him excerpts from the Tao Te Ching.

"Really?" I ask, "You don't hear the meaning in it?"

He doesn't.

He is hearing it for the first time. What did I expect? Even after years of dog-earing it, this ancient writing can be as cryptic as a *New Yorker* cartoon. (You know how some *New Yorker* cartoons are highbrow but you get them, you laugh, and others are higher-than-your-brow? Same with the Tao Te Ching.) Some of its verses still change shape right before my eyes.

"The Tao that can be told is not the eternal Tao," one translation reads. How am I supposed to *tell* it then? To discuss it? I have this idea to explore and write about these teachings, I think they can help.

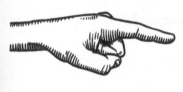 And that is when an image of a pointer finger flashes before me. Sitting in my dark kitchen in the middle of the night, I keenly understand the purpose of my work. You see, that is what this book is—the original one, as well as my own current guidebook—it is a pointer to a truth that already resides within us. *This way*, it gestures, *turn your head, alter your perspective, peel back the labels.*

Such a return, such a shift in one's thinking is the most easeful of tricks, like inhaling a breath of fresh air—but at times, it feels like a death. It is a spiritual experience that's as paradoxical as the text itself, unnerving even. Haven't most of us worked so hard to solidify our armor, along with our tenuous existence? Yet the Tao Te Ching clearly reveals its transience—which is why I scrambled to re-read it when the Coronavirus pandemic hit. I yearned for revelations, and I finally got 'em.

Many of us now understand how frail our manmade reality is. Like a set in a film of sorts, it only looks real. Careers, possessions, a filled-up calendar, *Don't overvalue these constructs,* the Tao keeps whispering. Better to learn to exist through comfort and discomfort alike. I hadn't always known that and I still need regular reminders. And life grants them to me, as it does to all of us—with a smack.

Still, no matter what happens, we can find ease by surrendering. "Accept what is and go from there," I've taken to saying—rather than raging or escaping or ignoring what you don't like. Everything we need to thrive is already here, underneath the bullshit. We already *are* the people we are hoping to become. We always were.

Naming the Nameless

"Names that can be named must change with time and place," the Tao preaches, reminding us that what you call a thing—tomato, tomahto, *pomidor* in Russian—doesn't define the thing itself.

"No matter how much we monogram it," I want to add, as I glance upon my kids' inscribed towels and blankets—all gifts commonly given at birth. But babies cannot even grasp the idea of their own individual personhood, let alone the name we choose for them after painstaking deliberation; they exist in a state of oneness. They *are* their hungry tummy, their mother's breast, the air, the sunlight, each other. So we begin to instruct them, labeling everything they see and touch, unwittingly teaching them separateness. This endless stream of titles and classifications may help their brains arrange the world before them, and yet, it is not the world.

My own given title—my birth name, Asya—despite being an arbitrary construct, brought me a lot of grief in my young life. It set me apart in America, as heavy and solid as a brick, just like my accent.

"Aszhha?" my teachers would ask on the first day of school after squinting at their attendance sheet. Or, "Ass-ya," they'd call out with confidence, as other kids snickered.

"Ahh-see-ya nothing in your chest," one creative classmate chanted. I'm not sure how I can still hear his sing-songy voice so clearly; I guess that's because it hurt. It seems small now, but it felt like my entire life at the time. I changed my name to Jessie when I entered high school, determined to get a fresh start, a new identity. I changed a lot of things.

It took me a couple decades to make my way back to the good, somewhat abandoned parts of Asya—the confidence, the curiosity, the unbridled joy with which I came into this world, and then this country—my essence. I think of these pieces as Asya, the me I left behind and then picked up again, but of course . . . tomato, tomahto, *pomidor*.

I now watch my daughters take a lot of pride in their first and middle monickers. Having never had a middle name myself—no one did where I came from—I wanted my kids to enjoy the way theirs rolls off the tongue, even if it's only while they're little and impressionable. What they like, I think, is how the entire first, second, third title gives them a shiny calling card and holds space for them. Perhaps that's what I had been after too, what we are all after.

Yet by learning to turn off our ever-working minds for just a moment, we set ourselves free. Instead of naming, categorizing, and sorting the world around us, we grow spacious. We lose our names, and gladly. This might be a split-second experience, or it can feel timeless. If we're lucky, we get to enter through the doorway of all understanding. We begin dwelling in the mystery of existence, and, gradually, then all of a sudden, we are swept up by its current—we are one with the Tao.

Within this energy, we transcend everything that distracts and drains us, including the limited boxes in which we've placed ourselves. Many spiritually inclined folks are able to do this by meditating. Adam goes running. Others do yoga, or paint, dance, or commune with nature. You don't even need to define it; like, I'm not sure what I do specifically anymore. I feel like 90 percent of my life is spiritual devotion at this point. I read, write, and listen to inspiring words, I pet my cat, swing into the treetops with my kids, I fight, I chill with pot and candles and crystals, I make up, I try to do, be, feel better.

I'm not saying that you should be like me or like anyone else; the Tao surely never says that. I'm saying you should be like *You*—the real You that's beyond the noise—whether you commit to it for moments a day or entirely. It's time to stop running from the unknown as if it will eat you alive (it may, actually—but it will only eat away at the facade or the ego). Instead, let's make room for the mystery. It can transform us if we let it.

Do Your Tao

Find some sort of flora or fauna, or a person that is extremely familiar to you—I'm choosing my old cat for this exercise, while he's curled up on the couch. Take a few moments to sit quietly and look at this sleeping child, this tree, this animal. Just watch them breathe in and out or sway in the breeze. Watch them and forget what they are called, what they represent. Truly observe and see the Universe, God, Tao, the life force in this object. The magic you witness in them is also in you, as it is in everyone—the names we give, the categorization, the separation are all an illusion.

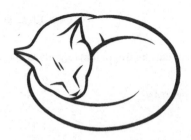

2

"I Love You," "I *Not* Love You"

People see beauty in what they call "beauty,"
that way they know of the "ugly."
People see good in what they call "good,"
that way they know of the "bad."

Existence and emptiness are concepts that make sense by
     comparison:
long lends meaning to short, and high to low.
But harmony is produced when sounds combine in unison;
before and after arrive as one.

Thus the Master acts without action and teaches the unspoken
     teaching.
Things arise and she lets them come.
Things disappear and she lets them go.
She lives openly with apparent duality and paradoxical unity.
When her work is done she forgets it,
that is why it lasts forever.

—TAO TE CHING, VERSE 2

As my then-two-year-old bluntly put it in regards to her sister,

"I love baby, I not love baby."

Accepting the Paradox

The reality we inhabit is always changing. We understand this on some level, which is why we often live in fear. We torture ourselves when life is going smoothly in anticipation of losing what we've got, and then again as we buck against the loss itself. So, weirdly, the collective other shoe dropping in 2020 ushered in emotional relief for some of us—we, the anxious, depression-prone types, may have been more alone physically, but we felt more unified psychically. Also, losing the control we'd tried to hold on to so tightly? I'm still not sure what it felt like . . . perhaps, inevitable?

One day in the midst of the pandemic, as my husband sat home without work and my bewildered children fought over a stupid toy, heavy rain and wind blasted our little town, bringing down trees and electric wires. When our power went out, we dug up flashlights and candles—even our menorah for posterity. We forced ourselves to take a neighborhood walk in the aftermath. Everything looked and smelled heavenly, surreal in its post-storm quietude. Lost in thought, I skipped over rocks—until I slipped and tumbled down like a clumsy bear cub, smashing my shin into an amorphous swollen trunk every shade of blue and purple. As the pain coursed through my bone, I threw myself back against the still-wet cement road and laughed hysterically. My family thought I had lost my mind but in that moment, I was the sanest I'd been in weeks. In my literal downfall, I felt a profound surrender—a peace that had been lacking in our joint state of grief and fear.

I get it, Universe, I thought, *I get it*, not even understanding what exactly it was that I was getting. I hobbled home and wrapped a cold towel around my leg and then assembled dinner by candlelight. I fell into a dreamless sleep that night as I stopped fearing the loss of all that's good in my life, and instead, wearily embraced the present.

"Life is like a zebra," my dad once told me, "dark lines are followed by white ones and vice versa." *Feel the pain, but look for the light,* is what I think he was telling me through his cheery buzz.

He was comforting me after my wrought, dramatic teenage break-up. "You can never regret what you did," he also said, "only what you didn't do." It was late at night after one of my parents' many get-togethers, where ex-Soviets partied with Soviet gusto—dancing in close quarters, singing, debauchery, kinship. I used to intermittently hide in my room when mom and dad threw one of their crowded bashes. The long parties beloved by my community were a bit much for my own sensibilities—too much food, perfume, alcohol, noise—but I enjoyed joining them in their off-kilter aftermath, when they bestowed life truths upon me.

Well, in this verse of the Tao Te Ching, Lao Tzu reminds us that being and non-being create each other. It is because of the noise that I sought out quietude. It's because of my heartbreak that I yearned for peace. When I came to the United States and felt displaced, I longed for connection. When I was distraught and bulimic, I wanted health; deep in depression, I needed a miracle.

The same is true of everyone. If you reflect on the various periods of your life, you will see how your messes gifted you with wisdom or resilience, how the before brought you to the after.

Ironically, it's in the low points that we often surrender to life's mysteries.

. . . .

being and non-being
create each other

. . . .

Embracing Duality

Very young children are able to grasp the reality of our dualistic existence better than we do.

"I like baby and I don't like baby," my older daughter, then two, would say about her little sister. "I love you; I not love you," the little sister would later echo to the older one. And more recently, "I love Charlie *and* I hate Charlie," adding, "but more love" on a good day.

Don't we all feel that way? Paradoxical in our emotions, mixed up in our identity, vision, and belief systems.

How do we live with this duality, then, without getting sucked into one end or the other? How can we find truth and balance amidst the polarity?

I've always wanted to be a spiritual, enlightened person but I never actually felt like one. Deep down, my thoughts could be very far from godly. Since rediscovering the Tao, though, I have been able to reframe my self-appraisal:

I am enlightened, I realized, *and* I act like a petty toddler.

I am friendly and sweet, *and* I can be judgmental.

I am supportive of other people, *and* I have pangs of jealousy.

The beauty of the Tao Te Ching is that it gives us permission to be many things at once. It is impossible to be perfect in our flawed, human world. Once we realize this and accept it, we can be a little less hard on ourselves, our children, and everyone around us.

I love my husband and I long for solitude.

I am a devoted mother and I get fed up with my kids.

My children mean everything to me *and* I know they are not mine; they came here with their souls fully loaded, ready to live and light up the world, and fail and make mistakes, and, hopefully, get back up again, though even that is not for me to decide. They feel like they belong to me right now, nuzzling into my neck like sweet puppies, but this is just a moment in time. I try to savor it as best I can (I also hide in the bathroom when needed).

I'm well aware the kids will grow and fly off one day. And I will let them. My heart will break for a minute. Still, I will give them the space to flourish. To have without possessing is the true definition of love—to open your arms when they need you and to release them when they do not—this is the blueprint, this is the lesson.

As things arise, let them come; as things disappear, let them go.

Do Your Tao

Pick a few areas in your life where your feelings or beliefs are conflicted: write down your jumble of messy thoughts or discuss them with a partner—and then let yourself be exactly who you are, denying nothing, owning everything.

Right now, for example, as I write this amidst lockdown, filled to the brim with sad stories and an unclear future, I am letting myself be both solemn and anxious, and ready to welcome a societal shift. I'm both grateful and tired, excited and scared, cynical and hopeful. And, just ask Adam—I'm a spiritual guide who has moments of being anything but.

"You're not spiritual at all," he jabbed at me when I cursed during a recent fight, in front of the kids no less. And yet I am.

Let us allow ourselves to be as we are: beautiful, ugly, complex, simple, spiritual, human—and then let's release it all, the entire paradoxical burden of existence, if only for this moment.

Let us sleep soundly tonight.

3

The Tao of Mom

Heaven and Earth are impartial,
they make no distinctions.
The Sage too doesn't take sides;
he gives without condition.

The space between Heaven and Earth is like a bellows:
empty yet infinitely capable.
The more it is used, the more it produces.
The more you talk of it, the less you comprehend.

Sit quietly and find the truth within.
Hold on to the center.

—TAO TE CHING, VERSE 5

And, as I discovered upon becoming a mother:

Keep changing them diapers, and you won't even realize
you're doing it.
In many an undertaking, exhaustion gives way to delight and
vice versa—an endless cycle—
hold on to the center.

Tapping In

The more the Tao is used, the more it produces; the more you do something, the greater you get at it. We can tap into this positive spiral (the better it gets, the better it gets, in other words) until we eventually become the Tao in action.

Think of any creative undertaking: painting, writing, composing music—when it reaches magical levels, the person doing it is basically a channel—a bellows, "empty yet infinitely capable." Anything else done impeccably, be it running an operation, playing basketball, or doctoring, is also a Tao-like endeavor. Whenever I watch my physician mom in her element, I see her become one with her knowledge, her ability to diagnose, and to offer healing; she is confident and in control and seemingly inexhaustible. She is God-like to her patients, several of whom display her photo near their most prized religious relics as if she were a saint. After a long day in the office, though, when she leaves her state of flow, she is exhausted and human like the rest of us, neuroses and all. I used to covet the perfect, all-knowing mom the patients got, until I realized that so much of being a mother is about being imperfect but doing it anyway—simply showing up over and over and over again, like mine did, whether you are broken or whole or somewhere in between.

When I was about to become a mama myself, which I felt was my strongest calling, I was as nervous as any first-timer. I had a weirdly shaped uterus—heart-shaped actually—kind of sweet, but constraining; just ask Charlie, she swears she was uncomfortable in my tummy. Once I was put on bed rest due to its complications, Adam and I couldn't remain in our tiny fourth-floor walk-up in the city. I wasn't sure I wanted to leave Manhattan, but my ambivalence didn't last long.

Late one morning as I sat home alone typing away on my computer, a shadowy figure appeared behind the curtain of my bedroom window. *Plop* went the air conditioning unit, tumbling onto the floor as the shadow jumped in.

I sprung off the bed, ran to the kitchen, and grabbed a butcher knife holding it in front of my pregnant belly. Thankfully, upon seeing my weird warrior pose, the shadowy figure ran off . . . or tried to. He couldn't quite master the lock on my front door so I had to step in and open it for him: *Here Mr. Burglar, out you go.* It was more of a sitcom-style attempted robbery than a thriller. Still, it was all I needed to flee at warp speed.

After the break-in, Adam and I moved in with my parents in the burbs while searching for a home of our own. Soon, my old filial bedroom accommodated the two of us, along with our tiny five-pound daughter who demanded my sore breast on the hour. It had been a tumultuous pregnancy, the mental and hormonal effects of which I'd failed to take into account, as did everyone around me. That's the thing about postpartum depression—we hear of it but we don't expect to experience it. We anticipate the much preferred motherly bliss of our dreams.

The day me and baby left the hospital, seventy-two hours after my C-section, my folks attempted a celebratory feast with champagne. (Have I mentioned? The Russian culture is filled with celebratory feasts.) But my insides felt like hot coals. I wanted to crawl under the covers and never come out.

"Why is baby crying?" mama would ask.

"Why are you crying?" wondered Adam, exasperated. When I wasn't crying, I was lashing out.

I read parenting books and listened to a cacophony of advice, but for months I wasn't quite getting it. I felt more like a rag than a mother. I couldn't see past a sleep-deprived, hormone-induced darkness.

Thankfully, with the help of antidepressants and sleep-training, I started to come out of my fog. At my core resided an innate power to nurture and when I tapped into it, I was off and running. It was a universal power, God power, Tao power, and it was infinitely capable. *I* became infinitely capable.

Hour by hour, day by day, I took care of Baby Charlie. At first I was pretty isolated. Then as we moved into our new neighborhood, I met an entire community of moms, helping me feel normal. But the relationship between me and my child was built in those quiet moments when we taught each other how to be mother and daughter. The more I mothered, the more natural it felt, not the other way around. My rocky start was as it should have been. It forced me to find my center.

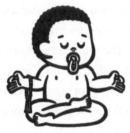

Let's add another kid to the mix, I thought, and so came Gigi Sweetie, as she dubbed herself.

Parenting is in my bones now. Like an artist who can paint with her eyes closed, I can console, advise, and retrieve missing toys in my sleep. At the end of the day, I'm a tired but happy husk.

Staying Neutral

Whenever I reconnect with the center which motherhood helped me uncover, I'm sort of able to channel that Taoist Sage—the one that doesn't take sides, the one that welcomes everything, the one that lives like the Tao itself. I mean, I'm not actually sure if these kind of

Sages or Masters exist among us mortals, but I *think* they make their earthly appearance once in a while. The rest of us, though, need only to aspire to this impartiality.

While I haven't evolved beyond my human faults and proclivities, when I swipe them out of the way, the Master is able to come through. So, even if I often fall short, it's my occasional mastery that I hope will shape my children—or rather will allow the Tao to shape them naturally, with minimal interference from my baggage.

My girls are best friends but also fierce competitors, and not taking sides can be easier said than done. I used to automatically protect my younger daughter—the baby—when she and my older one fought. Then I switched to shielding the older one, who seemed more distraught, more vulnerable. Yet, when I began to restrain myself, I observed the different ways that each girl negged her sister. I also found that if I floated in, said a few conciliatory words and retreated, they'd figure it out on their own.

They both know how to be kind and less than kind to one another. It is my job to love them through each side of the coin and to not favor "the good" over "the naughty" one or "the troubled" over "the stable" kid—labels that switch constantly. In every person there are so many different possibilities, which, after all, are only mirages. The Master sees past the illusion.

On a larger scale, this impartiality is even harder to accomplish. As I write this, our country is deeply divided—liberals versus conservatives, globalists versus nationalists, pro- and anti-quarantiners, and so on.

"Hold on to the center," the Tao instructs us. Give without condition.

Can we see the goodness underneath the discord, even if we have to dig and keep digging? Is it possible to find our way back to each other, despite our opposing views?

First, we must heal the discord within ourselves.

Do Your Tao

Choose a situation in your life where you feel you were treated unfairly or badly or when things just didn't go the way you wanted them to. Sit with the feelings for a moment and then think of or write down everything you learned from that situation or gained by dealing with it. Did it make you realize you're stronger than you thought? Did you need to become more resourceful or overcome your fear? Can you see the good on the other side of the bad? Find your center beyond the bad and good, past the pain, anger, and disillusionment. Bring yourself back to this center over and over again, regardless of what is going on around you. And when you fuck up — or feel fucked, for that matter — bring yourself right back there again, no matter how many tries it takes.

4

We're All the Great Mother
(Men, Too)

The Tao is known as the Great Mother;
empty yet inexhaustible, it is immortal.
It is like a vapor, barely seen but always present.
You can use it any way you want.

—Tao Te Ching, Verse 6

Or

To nurture, to rear, to renew—this is the Great Mother's power,
and it's at your disposal whenever you choose.
(Bonus: throw yourself into it wholly once in a while and you'll
get a break from ego.)

The Mother's Obliteration

"You need to get used to the fact that your time doesn't fully belong to you anymore," my best friend coached me when Charlie was first born, "You will create a new normal."

Despite a rocky start, I eventually did just that, settling into my all-encompassing role and reveling in it. I embraced the simplicity of temporary non-existence. I gave myself wholly to my babe, with her endless rolls and mischievous eyes. I lived to serve her: feed, bathe, stimulate, soothe, wipe bottom—not necessarily in that order.

No longer preoccupied with what I looked like, I exercised when she napped so I'd have the energy for an endless cycle of chores. We took walks, even in the freezing cold so she would get fresh air. I let her drink all the breastmilk she wanted as I watched *The Wire*, and made her smile and laugh, thus recharging my soul.

I grew calm, at peace, bottomless.

This freedom from my own needs, my own ego left a permanent imprint: a magical moment when time stood still and flew by simultaneously. I tried to replicate it when my second daughter was born, though then, it lasted but days. I had an older child and a community at that point. The blank slate was never to be repeated again.

As the girls have gotten older, I've reclaimed my identity—I aim to take care of myself, my relationships with others and with the world at large, along with caring for my children. A sprinkle of unavoidable mom guilt completes the picture. It is as it should be; I don't want to just disappear. Yet, in those early stages of motherhood, I felt closer to the Tao (God, the Universe) than ever.

At one point, I was contemplating having a third child just to experience the obliteration of self once more, not to mention my love of babies.

"No!" my husband stated with certainty, "we are so done."

"But are we really?" I kept wondering. Then I remembered the bed rest, the dreaded cerclage I had to get in my second pregnancy, the unavoidable C-sections to take my breached little beings out of my weird uterus. I thought of how our life is filled to the brim now—rambunctious children, a cat, projects, and aspirations, and of how challenging it is at times to get just two through the day in one piece.

"No," I agreed somewhat sadly, "no more babies for us it seems."

Still, if I close my eyes and sit quietly, I can feel the oneness I'd experienced with my newborn and with everything around us. I'm taken back to the power and beauty of my singular purpose, the inexhaustible giving, the joy of existence itself.

I miss that period of my life. I will always miss it. And that's okay.

The Mother's Immortality

"A mother has no age," the rabbi said as a masked handful of us buried my grandma, my dad's mama, in Queens during the spring of the pandemic. The next day, a friend lost her mom to COVID-19 after weeks of battling the illness.

"A mother has no age," I kept hearing on a loop. I thought of my small nearly hundred-year-old *babushka*, who'd lived countless lifetimes. Born in Moldova, she had to drop out of college to run from the Nazis, hiding in Uzbekistan and working in a plane factory until it was safe to return. She then married and dedicated her life to her kids and grandkids, following them to America.

God, she must have grown sick of reinventing herself.

Still, a mother has no age, a mother is always needed. At least that's what it feels like to me now, when I can't go a minute without "Mom" being yelled out by one of my kids.

"Mom, mama, mommmy!" and so forth.

But what do you do when your mom is gone? Or when she can't be approached because of some killer virus? What can you do when you didn't get to properly say goodbye?

Rather than tending to her own pain, my friend worried about her children—how to tell them about their lost grandmother, how to console them. "A mother never stops worrying for her children," the rabbi had said. "You can continue to ask her for guidance even after she's passed." A mother never rests, it seems.

I headed to the grocery store to purchase some flowers and a card, for whatever it was worth—a piece of paper that couldn't possibly relay the sorrow I felt on my friend's behalf. The sympathy card section had been pillaged, minus a few cheesy stragglers and some empty envelopes left behind. *Strange*, I thought. When I searched the greeting card aisle at the pharmacy, it too was short on bereavement cards. With the sight of yet another empty card holder, I finally got it: how many caskets had crowded the funeral home the day before, how many cards were needed. I reached for the only remaining option. All of a sudden, I wanted my mommy.

we are all longing to be mothered

We were all longing to be mothered then (we still are)—we, America, we, the world. We wanted our mamas to tell us it will be okay, that our children will be okay, that this too shall pass. We needed cuddles and comforting words and warm cups of tea or milk or whiskey. But even those of us lucky enough to still have moms couldn't get this sort of comfort. We were afraid to get too close, afraid to share the same air with the ones who'd raised us.

What then, could we do in lieu of the motherly touch? Phone calls, sure—if you had a parent to call. Maybe socially distant visits and air hugs. But then what?

I thought of the way the Tao Te Ching presented the Great Mother as a kind of feminine energy available to all of us. We were all born of her and we could also use her power as we wished—her regenerative force, that renewal we'd been craving.

It was time, I realized, to dig deep and find the Great Mother—the Tao—within ourselves.

The Mother Within

I get the Tao because I *was* the Tao for a brief period. But you don't have to be a parent to experience it for yourself. You just need to let go of your own worldliness, with all of its baggage, needs, and ambitions. For just a moment a day, drop it like a heavy suitcase. Imagine not being the complicated you, but still being—an awareness, a simple, pervasive existence—the greater You.

"To know yourself as the Being underneath the thinker, the stillness underneath the pain, is freedom, salvation, enlightenment," wrote spiritual philosopher Eckhart Tolle in *The Power of Now*. He said in our modern-day world, we all tend to overthink and over-plan, spending so much time in wanting that we miss out on the joys of being. But we can change that!

Do not be afraid to lay down your load for a minute. You can pick it up again any time you wish. Separate yourself from your endless goals and grievances. It will recharge you like nothing else. Spend a breath, then two, then an hour flowing without worry and doing what needs to be done without overthinking it, and bask in existence itself. This is the ultimate freedom.

Since we are but human, it is not a state we can remain in indefinitely. I constantly find myself sliding back towards worldly ambition or a bottomless need for something, anything, everything. What I can do (what you can also do) is bring myself back, reminding myself of the "being underneath the thinker." That way, when I run around in this paper world like a wound-up toy, I remember that somewhere within me, the Great Mother—with her heart-shaped uterus—resides. Everything else is but noise.

Do Your Tao

Are you a mother or a father? An aunt, a friend, or a pet parent? Find something or someone who needs nurturing and give yourself over to this mothering completely. It doesn't have to be a long exercise, but for whatever length of time you choose—be it a half-hour or a day—commit yourself to caring for a person, an animal, or a plot of land. Make your own needs secondary for this period and focus all your power on another living thing. Enjoy the state of giving; enjoy a break from your human self. (Plus: for all the parents out there, this giving-over—being all mom or all dad for an hour, or even for fifteen minutes when that's all you've got—benefits your connection with your children greatly.)

5

Off the Leash

Can you concentrate your mind and soul until you return to the
*   original oneness?*
Can you keep your breath soft and smooth, just as an infant would?
Can you love people and lead them without forcing your will on
*   them?*
Can you step back from your own understanding
and thus understand all things?

Giving birth and nourishing,
creating without possessing,
acting with no expectations,
leading without trying to control . . .
This is the mysterious virtue.

—TAO TE CHING, VERSE 10

So,

Can you tell your inner busy body to take a hike and instead go
take one yourself?

Grasping

Our world can be a difficult place to focus. Increasingly difficult, as we are bombarded by constant stimuli and the ever-present news cycle. In our daily life, we often find ourselves busy, busy, busy—with our jobs, our children, our plans. "So busy," "So tired," is a badge of honor. But in the dark, many of us can't stop our monkey-minds from spinning.

I once thought the demands of modernity are what keep us from peace. Yet, even as normal life came to a halt in 2020, our endless activities and planning were simply replaced by worry. Plus, we found ways to overstimulate ourselves anyway.

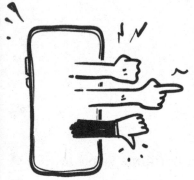

Who hasn't spent half the night doomscrolling or tried to read an article, a book, and Twitter all at once, while concurrently texting? A good way to achieve very little and to doze off way too late, waking up less than refreshed in the morning. And, look, it's okay, but let's at least be self-aware—so it's a conscious choice to embrace a state of entropy.

On the other hand, when we reach for flow (see chapter 22), moments, minutes, hours fly by in a blink as we get lost in one specific task. We are off somewhere else, swimming in the words or the moves or the art coming through us, or absorbed by the simple rhythm of walking, biking, petting an animal. Those moments, that energy, help us balance out the chaos.

"Can you concentrate your mind and soul until you return to the original oneness?" Lao Tzu asked. My answer is, "Sometimes. Not often enough. I'm working on it."

My personality is that of a busy body. I want to know everything, judge and categorize everyone, anchor myself with my thoughts, my decrees, my temporary grasp on the world. But there's also a greater, eternal Me, which sits above all of it. It is aligned with the original oneness the Tao Te Ching speaks of—a dimension where all is still, even as the world whirls by. Our busy reality fades away, and I am in tune with God, the Universe, the Tao.

It is from that place that great things happen.

Letting Them Be

When it comes to the bonds with our significant others, our children, friends, family, and whoever else is meant to cross our path, the Tao asks, "Can you love people and lead them without forcing your will?"—without controlling, without possessing, without expectations, even?

It's a lot to ask.

It is also the definition of unconditional love.

We've all glimpsed the benefits of letting people be as they are. I notice with friends, when I show kindness and support without expectations, that is often what comes back to me, even if it's from a different source. And I know the best way to lead is to shine my own light so that those who see it feel a sense of permission to do the same. I know this because that's how I found my permission—by basking in the bright light of others.

With my husband, I've learned that if I am upset, I need to look at myself—where am I withholding whatever I seek from him? Of course, just because I understand this doesn't mean I do it. We sometimes need to peel off the layers of resentment with pliers—#marriagelife, am I right? Still, if I feel underappreciated, I often notice I too am not showing enough appreciation. When he is playing tit-for-tat with all the duties of running a household, I recognize that I've been doing the same, at least in my head. Once I pivot, though, allowing him to be who he is without any conditions, I bring ease into our relationship. Not demanding, I want for nothing, fully valuing all he is and does. In freeing him, I free myself.

And in raising daughters, I aspire to nourish them wholly—
flaws, feelings, and all. It is also what I am trying to do for myself.
Because I cannot lead my girls in being free and full if I don't embody these very traits. I cannot properly lead anyone that way. None
of us can.

Do Your Tao

Treat your relationship with yourself as the primary model for all
the relationships in your life. Give yourself the acceptance and
enhancement you seek. Focus on where you got it right, rather than
beating yourself up for what you got wrong; compliment yourself
more, criticize less. When you feel dejected, boxed in, uninspired,
don't force yourself to do anything. Let go of all the worldly rules
and constraints and step out of the matrix to gain perspective. Then
take yourself out of yourself entirely. Dissolve.

I get there via nature, writing . . . sometimes meditation. How
are you gonna do it?

6

"F*ck This, I'm Water"

The supreme good is like water,
for water benefits all things and goes against none of them.
It provides for all and even cleanses those places a man is
  loath to go.
Therefore, it is like the Tao.

Live in accordance with the nature of things:
make where you live a good place,
make your mind a mind of depth.
Give your benevolence indiscriminately to others.
Speak the truth, govern well, work well to set into motion the
  good times.

Such is the way to live without contention.
Such is the man free from complaints and anguish.

—TAO TE CHING, VERSE 8

And remember,

You, yourself, are mostly water. Flow on!

Watering

When I was in my twenties, going through one of my many dramas, I turned to my chiller, smarter brother for guidance.

"Be like water," he told me, "just roll over shit and say, 'Fuck this, I'm water.'"

And when this same brother was holed up in his Brooklyn apartment, recovering from COVID—and I was living one long day at a time in the suburbs as my kids' teacher, cook, playmate—his words became my soundtrack.

I'm water, I mumbled to myself repeatedly. *I. Am. Water.*

The funny thing is, when he first gave me this suggestion to emulate liquid, I brushed it away like a crumb. I was not interested enough in stillness or inner peace, which were pretty much the opposite of my then chaotic existence. I was always suffering in those years—a whirlwind of ecstasy and pain—giving my power away to whoever would take it: any guy I fell for, who inevitably treated me like crap, or, at best, ignored me, or to some leering talent manager who told me I wasn't beautiful but at least I was sexy.

"Here you go, here's my power," I'd practically belt out on my knees, "make me a star or a girlfriend; make me something that matters."

Of course, no one else had the capability to fix my life. Only I did.

And when my stupid, often self-created circumstances did in fact look like a pile of excrement, my brother was right—it was time to roll over it and flow on. So eventually, that is what I did.

Here's the thing: water itself *is* the savior. It is ever-transforming, ever-sustaining and it's boundless. In this way it is just like the Tao, like God. And we, too, can aim to be Tao-like. The human body, after all, is made up of mostly H_2O.

As Bruce Lee famously said in the 1970s TV show *Longstreet*:

You must be shapeless, formless, like water. When you pour water in a cup, it becomes the cup. When you pour [it] in a bottle, it becomes the bottle . . . Water can drip and it can crash. Become like water my friend.

This liquid also nourishes everything it comes in contact with, not caring if you are rich or poor, good or bad, flora or fauna; it cleanses you and keeps you alive. Practicing such non-judgement is the ultimate Tao. That's the benevolence we witness in doctors and nurses, firemen, teachers, neighbors, janitors—it emerges in every scope and walk of life.

But as I, too, tried to step up to what the moment asked of me, I sometimes found myself falling short. I got agitated with my freewheeling children, I resented my constantly hungry husband, I cursed politicians left and right. I bucked the flow, feeling the anxiety constrain my chest (or was it COVID-19?!).

Thankfully, though, I'd been a student of the Tao since my misguided youth. It had helped me through addictive, self-destructive behavior, and many an awful thought. And so I'd learned to accept my catty inner voice (when I tried to extinguish it, it only grew) and to let my emotions ping-pong every which way. Rather than get caught up in them, I allowed them to be and then to pass. I reminded myself that I can exist in both a dropper and in the ocean. Eventually, I gave in to the shape of whatever the situation called for. I cared for my children, I binge-watched *Tiger King*.

Because life had forced me to recalibrate before, and because this masterful philosophy had shown me how, I was able to find peace within me much of the time. When I couldn't, when I didn't know what to do, I stopped. I did nothing at all, other than wipe butts and break up fights—that one's my non-negotiable, especially with the children home all day, every day. But I was able to cease my constant planning and worrying and to wait. I knew if I could keep my mind still, the next step would become obvious. I streamed all of myself into the kiddie pool as needed, awaiting the day I'd be set loose to evaporate and to return as a goddamn thunderstorm, or post-pandemic dew or something.

You too know intuitively how to adjust and flow and vaporize. You too are a shapeshifter, more fluid than you may have realized.

And again, in the words of my brother: "Fuck this, I'm water."

Say it to yourself as often as needed.

Do Your Tao

For the next couple days, as you drink, shower, or bathe in water, pause to contemplate its nature. Mentally thank it for quenching your thirst and for washing you clean. As you go to sleep, think about its presence in your body (the average adult human body is 50-65 percent water). How can you emulate it in your day-to-day existence? Which situations in your life can benefit from more fluidity?

The next time you get worked up, remind yourself of your powerful liquid properties, and flow on.

7

Donuts, Crack, and Other Addictions

Overfill your cup and it will spill.
Sharpen a blade too much and it will chip off in use.
Fill your house with jade and gold and you will only bring
*   insecurity.*
Care about people's approval and you will be their prisoner.

Do your work, then step back—
the only path to serenity.

—TAO TE CHING, VERSE 9

Simply,

Know. When. To. Stop.

Compulsion

Any addict can sense what this verse is pointing to; those of us whose addictive side has been triggered can have trouble discerning when to stop. In this way, every addiction—be it food, pills, alcohol, shopping—is the same: the impulse for more, always more. But compulsively filling our hunger doesn't work. We get desperate and messy, until we are lying face down on the floor begging for mercy.

For seven years of my life I was bulimic. I gorged myself until my stomach distended like a balloon and then I puked it all up like the possessed little girl in *The Exorcist*—or like Princess Diana, as *The Crown* reminded us. I can't tell you how many hours of my existence I spent "overfilling my cup" and then expunging it, how many pounds of food I wasted. It is shameful. I've been well for over fifteen years and I still carry some shame. But, if I'm honest, I also get a thrill remembering how insatiable I once was.

"Did I ever tell you I used to eat a dozen donuts for breakfast and then throw them all up?" I asked Adam once.

"What? A whole dozen?" he balked. I'm five-foot-two and used to curl up in my daughters' cribs.

"Yes! And then a super-sized meal from Burger King."

"That's insane," he said.

"I know, right?" I exclaimed in triumph, "insane."

I get perverse pleasure from recalling the extent of my gluttony. It's easier to paint a caricature of myself: the small girl gobbling up huge quantities of food, than to talk about the pain. It was easier to be that caricature, in fact—the one who would sit in class thinking of what she would binge on on her way home—than to be a complex person with nondescript trauma who actually let herself feel what she felt.

Still, I am not sorry for having been sick in the head once. I will never forget praying to a nebulous god on the cold bathroom floor. The Tao, like water, flows to the bottom, to *our* bottom, to cleanse us. From my brokenness, I searched for healing. That was its purpose; I found my way, my Tao, in this search.

If you are reading these words, whether you are shattered or whole, the Tao is reaching for you as well.

Let it.

Moderation

Lao Tzu wrote about incorporating moderation into every part of our lives—in seeking pleasure, money, acclaim—knowing when to stop is key; not knowing when to stop can be our pitfall. What pleasure is there in the never-ending rat race? Not much. The sheen of the accolades is short-lived.

In Japan, hard work is lauded perhaps even more than American ambition and people are actually dying of it. The Japanese word *karoshi* translates as "death by overwork." Its medical cause is often heart attack or stroke, and some see it as a cultural crisis.

Too much of anything, be it work, drunken merriment, or exercise will wreak havoc. Thus, the Tao Te Ching advises us to find and create equilibrium, to balance the many facets of existence. Ask yourself which parts of your life you prioritize at the expense of other areas. How can you spread your energy out more evenly?

In my case—addictions aside—parenthood proved to be a challenge in poise. Upon becoming a mother, I dove all in. No more job, no more frivolity. I existed only to care for another. At first I imploded, and then I lost myself in it. Slowly, I've been rebuilding a multi-faceted self, with time away from my omnipresent mom duties (pandemic, notwithstanding). After all, a fulfilled parent in smaller quantities is far better than 100 percent of a discontented one—the same goes for any role in life.

I've also realized my little women need freedom to be their own developing selves instead of existing as their mother's *raison d'être*. I don't want to train them to constantly seek my approval, or anyone else's for that matter—I'd like for them, for all of us gals, to find it from within.

Do Your Tao

"Care about people's approval and you will be their prisoner," this text tells us. Stop giving a damn, or at least care less . . . it's such an exhausting preoccupation. And yet, it isn't always easy *not* to care. We are human creatures who seek connection. We want to not give a fuck, but we do.

If you find yourself overly concerned with the opinion of others, remember that real connection is different from approval—it's based on authenticity, which is not possible if you're constantly trying to satisfy or placate. As a recovering people pleaser (just another compulsion, by the way), I must remind myself of this regularly.

"Do your work, then step back," says the Tao Te Ching. Don't overanalyze who will like it and who won't. Don't fret so much about its results. Give your all as you're doing it and then stop. Allow yourself to feel a deep sense of satisfaction dependent on nothing and on no one outside of your own being.

8

Get in the Freaking Pool

Just as the colors that we see can blind us,
so the tones that we hear can deafen us,
and the flavors that we taste can dull our palate.

The chase and the hunt craze people's minds,
so goods that are difficult to get become hurdles in our life journey.

The Sage is led by his inner truth and not his outer eye.
He holds to what is deep and not what lies on the surface.

—Tao Te Ching, Verse 12

Similarly,

You can't feast on everything all at once (trust me, I tried),
and you can't look to everyone else for advice.
Stop keeping up with the Joneses;
listen to that little voice within.
Make up your own mind, friend.

The Paradox of Choice

I was just shy of eight years old as my family, seeking asylum in America, awaited our fate in Europe. We left the USSR, with its limited choices and lack of exposure to the outside world and set off to a land I knew nothing about. First we took an overnight train from my birthplace of Riga, Latvia, to Moscow. From Moscow we flew to Austria. There we were hoarded into an apartment with strangers—one room per family unit—nothing new, after spending years in a government-issued communal apartment. But when we exited this refugee holding pen, we were free to roam the streets of Vienna, which was beautiful, magical, and overwhelming. My dad took us to a pristine park. Everything felt and smelled crisp and fresh, unlike the stench of Soviet-era vehicles. An ice cream truck pulled up with its giant menu—pictures of frozen concoctions that blew my mind. I'm not sure how long it took me to make my choice; I simply remember clutching a bright green frog, licking it furiously so that not a drop would be lost.

Upon entering a European supermarket, my head spun. I had only ever been exposed to Soviet markets, many of their shelves empty; think quarantine, but all the time: a constant shortage of toilet paper. My parents, aunt, uncle, grandma, cousin—we were all floored by the colors of the free-world packaging and the sheer quantity of products. It felt like we'd been jetted from a black-and-white existence straight into technicolor.

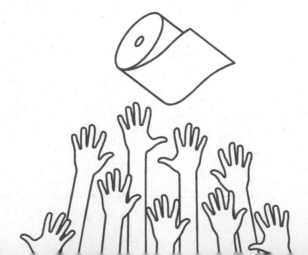

Oh the joy of mixing blueberry yogurt with sticky *Smacks* cereal (another frog, by the way, as the cereal's mascot; no clue why amphibians sang to me). In America, we feasted on Pop-Tarts and Entenmann's. Orange juice, apple juice, fruit punch. Endless hues and varieties of sugar.

After a while, the novelty wore off—but the need for more, sweeter, better remained. At one point, I owned too many clothes, too much makeup, too many pairs of uncomfortable shoes. I dressed myself up like a doll and secretly stuffed my face with junk. A pretty, dainty figurine, I clogged toilets with vomit everywhere I went. All the colors and flavors just masked my inner turmoil. Until I faced this struggle and explored it wholly, mine was a surface life.

Learning to live with choice rather than being overwhelmed by it is a vital lesson—much like learning to hear your inner guide in a cacophony of voices.

Choosing

One recent summer at a neighborhood pool party, I was the only woman in the pool.

"Good for you," said a local dad, amidst the other dads in the water, beers in hand. I plodded in deeper, submerging my low-grade discomfort.

How come the women didn't get in, while so many guys hung out there waist-deep, seemingly comfortable whatever shape they were in? Another mom came in soon after and I exhaled a sigh of relief without understanding why.

I get that I may have looked funny later, with my wet dress over my bathing suit, as a friend jokingly pointed out my soaked-through boobs. And the other ladies did maintain a well-coiffed, well-dressed look. Still, it was a hot day, I was cooled off, and I'd gotten to swim with my daughters. I hadn't set out to be different, though I do miss the memos sometimes. I guess I no longer care enough to heed them. I'm intent on showing my girls that women can and should have as much fun as men, that they can *be* as fun and as free. I'm intent on showing *myself.*

I simply decided to elevate my inner guide above the external din. Heeding this voice means being the one weirdo in the pool or rolling down a frozen hill with the kids or finding some other way to make a fool of yourself because it beats the constant adulting. But it can also mean saying "No." Just, "No." "No, thank you, I'm good." It's about going within rather than trying to keep up on the outside.

Do Your Tao

Guiding myself was an adjustment at first. Declining invitations felt uncomfortable, for example. I used to force myself to go to everything that was happening in my surroundings. I didn't ask myself if I actually wanted to. After all, I grew up in a community where there was always an occasion for festivities, with the endless food and the toasts. It was what you did. Not going was considered rude. But eventually the discomfort of doing what I didn't want to do became greater than the discomfort of going against the grain—the Russian grain, the American grain, it didn't matter.

If you, too, used to go places on autopilot, the shock of having the world stop must have been jarring. I invite you to mine that hardship for its gifts, inculding the beauty of a less-packed calendar.

While at first, the return of engagements and activities was a welcome rebirth, I think many of us felt overscheduled again very quickly. Let us take a pause now. Let's stop to inquire, "What makes me feel good? What makes me come alive?" and do more of *that*!

If it's connection, how can you bring a level of depth and authenticity into your relationships? If it's nature, if it's physical activity, if it's art, creation, spontaneity, solo time—make space for it. No need to limit yourself to what anyone else is doing; all choices can come from within—you have enough knowledge and agency to decide for yourself.

How frightening to stop asking those around us for advice, constantly curating opinions for every choice, every move. How freeing.

The Sage is led by his inner truth and not his outer eye.

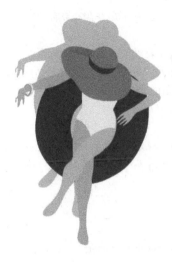

9

Virtue or Obligation?

When the greatness of the Tao is present, action arises from one's
*   own heart.*
When it is abandoned, righteousness appears.
If you need rules to be "kind" and "just," if you act virtuous,
this is a sure sign that virtue is absent.
Thus we see the great hypocrisy.

Only when the family loses its harmony do we hear of "dutiful sons."
Only when the country falls into chaos do politicians talk of
*   "patriotism."*

—TAO TE CHING, VERSE 18

Take it from a recovering pleaser:

Do it because you want to,
and if you really don't want to, don't do it!
Find your own brand of goodness—it's in there somewhere.

Do What You Want

Adam and I tend to shudder at the word "obligation." It's one of those intrinsic distastes that binds us together in a rather free life. We do most of what we do because we want to, with the regular obligations seeping in as they do. Whereas I can handle those compulsory social norms—I was once an obedient Soviet child, after all—Adam's crabbiness in response is almost comical.

"Why do we need to host?" he wants to know. "Why do we have to go to so-and-so's wedding? Do I have to wear pants? Why can't I get married in sneakers?"

It's as if he is allergic to rules. (He did get married in sneakers; April through October, he opts for shorts; and, abhorring large parties, his tendency is to hide in the bathroom.) At the same time, the guy's a devoted husband and father, a hard worker, a loyal friend. His commitment comes from the heart, rather than from external instruction: for example, since he is constantly bucking authority, he thrives as a freelancer—he gets to be his own boss. He loves his kids more than anything in the world and finds time with them to be fun, fulfilling, and, yes, exhausting. Still, it's what he *wants* to be doing and he does it well.

"You are so Taoist," I wink at him.

"Extremely," he answers, and flows on.

But in reality, there are plenty of instances when everyone needs to do the things they don't initially find appealing or sincere, even. Then what?

For me, the answer is pausing. I wait until I can find and feel the positivity of what's being asked of me. And I say "No" if I cannot. I try do so kindly; perhaps I offer too many excuses and apologies— but for an ex-people pleaser, it's a start.

Another trick is focusing on what needs to be done *today*, rather than dreading something down the line. This way, future anxiety is alleviated, and more often than not, we can find a sliver of surprising enjoyment, even in what we usually deem unenjoyable.

My current existence is centered around my brood—the tiny beings I made that rely on me, entertain me, and drive me nuts—and their stubborn kid of a father. I am also part of a wider community, a larger family, a vast planet. Caring about children, animals, the Earth feels like alignment to me. So does being neighborly or checking on my grandmother, or simply connecting with the energy of all.

I try to spend my time in ways that bring me and others joy or fulfillment. From that perspective, obligations don't feel as such.

The more we search for the Tao, the more we find it within our own hearts—only from there can aligned action arise. Then rules, dutifulness, and also patriotism fade away.

The Tao of Trump

"Wake up, Trump has COVID," Adam announced the month before the 2020 election.

"Oh?" I said, not quite sure what to think as I opened my eyes.

After fully awakening (in my girls' bed . . . again) I understood why practically everyone I knew was so happy about the news. Strictly from a political standpoint, those of us who badly desired change saw his illness—after months of downplaying the pandemic—as his comeuppance. Yet, something in me stopped me from feeling gleeful.

I remembered how just a few years back, Donald Trump won his presidency with the motto, "Make America Great Again." He positioned his supporters as patriots and everyone else as the destroyers.

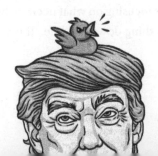

It worked; he had tapped into a deep divide and capitalized on it. And as vitriol from the left followed, it only added fuel to his fire. Folks ended friendships over this divisive man, families had blowout fights, my own included. Trump supporters were lumped in with Trump himself. As the years rolled on, the hatred increased— or perhaps it just rose to the surface.

Many of us felt angry, hurt, torn up by the behavior of this polarizing president, and our basic reaction was to lash out and to demonize all who supported him. What we didn't realize is that in so doing, we bought into the very divisiveness Trump had counted on to come to power. We simply added fuel to the inferno . . . for we inevitably become what we despise.

The Tao Te Ching warns of this "great hypocrisy"—the us-versus-them mentality. It forces us to recognize that despite our personal opinions, there are people of all political proclivities who are genuine. There are also tons of self-righteous hypocrites. These tendencies exist in everyone: we each carry goodness, as well as a shadow side. It is up to us to choose which energy to embody (not once, but time and time again).

"If you need rules to be kind and just, if you *act* virtuous, this is a sure sign that virtue is absent," says the Tao. How, then, do we find virtue within ourselves regardless of the rules, regardless of who is in charge?

I honestly don't know what the answers are. But thanks in part to my experiences as a Jew in the Soviet Union and then an unwelcome *Rusky* in post–Cold War American classrooms, I've gained the ability to find my center beyond labels. I am thankful for the present moment and for the possibility which it holds.

I wonder if anyone will ever run for president admitting they do not know how to alleviate our issues, but that they're willing to keep an open mind, "a beginner's mind," as they say in the East. Until then, I'll forever sip from the "Oprah 2020" cup my husband gave me. It was a gag gift because he finds my love of Oprah to be over the top. Nevertheless, a girl can dream.

Do Your Tao

In the realm of politics, our blood pressure is bound to spike. That is why it's so important to apply Taoist wisdom to help us stay calm amidst the political, economic, societal storms that are our reality. Feel good about your deepest beliefs and truths regardless of what you hear from others or see on the news. Remember that you don't need rules to be kind and just. Revel in the world's indomitable goodness and celebrate it wherever you see it. When you witness hypocrisy, understand it for what it is, but don't let it shake your core.

Have faith in yourself and in your connection to the Universe— when this connection is strong enough, no outer event can sever it. Every time you're about to lose your cool, find something beneficial you can do for another person, an animal, the planet, or your own spirit. The ripples of small virtuous acts are infinite.

10

Enough!

Abandon holiness and cleverness, and the people will benefit a
* hundredfold.*
Throw away righteousness, and people will do the right thing.
Discard schemes and profit-seeking, and people will not become
* thieves.*

These are outward forms alone, so I will add:
See with original purity,
embrace with original simplicity,
reduce what you have,
decrease what you want.

—Tao Te Ching, Verse 19

Basically,

Stop making people do things, including your children,
And, while you're at it, stop hoarding material possessions.
Just chill.

You Are Enough

"We are crazy monkeys," Charlie squealed into the dashboard as she and Gigi dialed everyone whose number popped up on my recently called list.

A few minutes before that, they were running in and out of an optics shop, trying on glasses and shrieking with delight.

"How old are they?" asked the sales clerk. Thankfully, she was amused rather than pissed off.

"Four-and-a-half and two-and-a-half," I replied on autopilot, sweating profusely.

I dragged them out of the store soon after, afraid they would break a pair of Chanel frames and leave me in debt—I'd come to this country with two-hundred dollars and still feared overspending.

As I was catching my breath, Gigi pressed the horn with her tummy, attracting the attention of an elderly passerby.

"Is everything okay?" she asked with concern after knocking on the window of my Toyota.

"Yes," I sputtered from the back, "Sorry, I'm just having trouble getting them in their car seats." In truth, I hadn't even tried yet.

"Oh, thank God," she said, "me and my girlfriend thought they were in there all by themselves . . ."

"Well, have fun," she added, backing away.

The thing is I was having fun. I mean I badly needed a shower, but while I often stammered and apologized for their cacophony, I'd secretly have a blast witnessing it. After I manhandled them into their seats, we went home and had a dance party. I fed them leftovers, washed the dirt off their squirmy little bodies, and wrangled them into bed.

These free-spirited daughters leave me spellbound and bone-tired. Clearly, I'm light on discipline—at least, for now.

"But how do you instill values in them?" my aesthetics-loving mama asked once, when I wouldn't force Gigi to change out of a soiled shirt. "How will they know what's dirty and what's clean, for example?"

"I don't really believe I need to instill very much," I shrugged.

Throw away righteousness, I thought, and people will do the right thing.

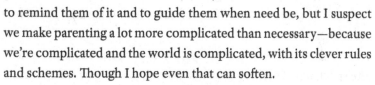

I feel keenly that all children have endless goodness within them. Sure, it is our job to remind them of it and to guide them when need be, but I suspect we make parenting a lot more complicated than necessary—because we're complicated and the world is complicated, with its clever rules and schemes. Though I hope even that can soften.

On the first day of kindergarten, Charlie came home with a letter from her teacher telling us that she encourages mistakes in class, how mistakes mean the kids are making an effort, that they're learning. "The same goes for adults," I read and reread, the Soviet child within me finally let off the hook. I realized these children might get at five what I understood at thirty-five: abandon holiness, embrace imperfection, you are enough.

You Have Enough

"Reduce what you have/Decrease what you want."
These words were written centuries ago. And now, in modern times, minimalism is a sort of trend—even here in the United States, perhaps the epicenter of consumerism. Practically everyone has tried Marie Kondo's "tidying up" technique—the one she demonstrates in her books and her Netflix series. "Does it bring me joy?" we ask ourselves before deciding what to keep and what to trash.

But long before her *KonMari* organizing method became a worldwide phenomenon, the man I was dating taught me the freedom of throwing shit out.

When you come from very little, like my family had, you tend to hold on to everything you acquire, despite eventually having more than you can handle. Many a person who lived through wars and starvation, like my grandma, later teetered on the verge of hoarding. My mom, who spent her Soviet youth with one dress and one pair of pants, in turn went gaga over all the lovely clothing in America—she'd purchase too much for herself, too much for me. And to this day, I find empty jars of fragrant moisturizers in her bathroom. I'm not sure what she's saving them for, just that it is hard for her to part with them.

When I met Adam, however, I was swept to the other side of the spectrum. Anything the dude doesn't use he gets rid of, including a perfectly good coffeemaker (he doesn't drink coffee) or an extra bottle of rubbing alcohol (except it wasn't rubbing alcohol; he threw away my peroxide). "I have a problem, I know," he jokes. He cannot stand clutter—one shirt in, one shirt out is his policy if he buys something new. It took me awhile to mostly align myself with this routine of purging closets and cabinets, and while, at times, he goes too far, I've embraced his habit of getting rid of material possessions—the freedom is enlivening.

Research shows materialism doesn't lead to satisfaction. And it's become clear that what people surround themselves with in their space is a reflection of their inner lives and vice versa. That being said, with two little kids, I simply settle for organized chaos—both within and without.

This is not a huge mess, I tell myself, taking in our LEGO-strewn living room. When I ask them to clean it up at night, they begrudgingly do—like, after the fifth request, with my help. And, I'll admit, we have too many Barbies: Barbies in the bath, on the stoop, practically everywhere I look is a tiny plastic creature. Recently though, Charlie began moving these dolls to Gigi's room. *A good start*, I thought. That's when she launched her campaign for OMG dolls—big sisters of the LOL dolls, in case you're not in the know.

In most kids' minds, there's no such thing as too many toys or too much candy. Mine are mesmerized by commercials and ads aimed to make them want everything under the sun. But my hope is that by example—and as they mature—they will learn that less is more and happiness cannot be bought, that the key is to enjoy exactly who they are, where they are, and what they have.

Do Your Tao

Bucking our consumerist culture of endlessly wanting and shopping can get us closer to the original purity written about in the Tao Te Ching. *Whenever you can, simplify*, it is telling us—simplify your thoughts, your plans, your possessions.

What can help you streamline your life?

Maybe you follow Marie Kondo's advice and get rid of any item that doesn't bring you joy: socks on the verge of holes, the shirt you never want to wear, the vase you hate but keep around anyway. Plus, the next time you feel the urge to make a purchase, pause; just pause for a moment to consider why you're buying the item.

Apply the same thought process to your plans and aspirations—*Will attending this bring me joy? Why do I want to achieve this?*—and watch both your outer and inner life untangle. Remember, peace lies beneath the clutter.

11

The Tao of *Babushka*

*If you can still the restlessness of the mind, the heart will be at peace;
you will see all living things around you in a new light.*

*Each separate being in the Universe returns to the common source;
returning to the source is tranquility.*

*To know the eternal process of return brings enlightenment.
To miss the process brings disaster.
When you realize where you come from, you naturally become
tolerant, disinterested, amused, kindhearted as a grandmother,
dignified as a king.
Immersed in the wonder of the Tao, you can deal with whatever life
brings you,
and when death comes, you are ready.*

—Tao Te Ching, Verse 16

Or

External life can be a crapshoot, but your inner life—it's all yours.
Seek out the light, even in the darkest of places, and peace even in
the most turbulent of times;
we all return to Source either way.

Curveballs

My grandmother Babushka Dina and I didn't always get along when I was young. We had lived together most of my childhood but once we immigrated, she became my nanny. Taking care of my little brother and me while our parents toiled to set up a life, she wasn't quite the kindhearted grandmother Lao Tzu refers to—not then anyway. She was tough. She had spent her adulthood as a respected math teacher, not a babysitter, and having led such a hard life, she had little patience for my modern entitlement.

She'd lived through the Holocaust, struggled for food, lost both her parents at a young age, as well as her partner.

"How come you never dated again?" I asked her once; she'd been widowed at forty-five.

"I had a husband, he died," she answered.

My grandfather—her husband—passed away alone in Siberia after Babushka and their children had moved back to her homeland of Latvia. Virtually all Jews were eradicated in Latvia during the Holocaust, including much of her family. When I asked her why she'd been so determined to go back, she simply said it was home—returning was always the plan.

Still, my grandfather, who quit school at thirteen when both his parents were sent to one of Stalin's labor camps, feared starting over. Twenty-five hundred miles away from his wife and kids, he built houses and chain-smoked, hoping to one day rejoin them. Babushka received his final letter *after* his fatal heart attack. He had almost secured a job in Riga, she told me—where I was eventually born.

"Thank you for having existed" was the phrase she chose for his tombstone.

Later in America, her son, my uncle, died of cancer. Her younger sister, whom she'd been separated from for decades, passed away as well. Many of her friends bit the dust.

This all sounds very depressing, I know, trust me—and she knows. And yet, Babushka found a way to soften into her role, now as the kindhearted great-grandmother who spoils my girls with too much chocolate. Prior to the pandemic, she enjoyed Silver Sneakers—an exercise program for seniors, as well as Yiddish classes, and she'd whizz throughout Brooklyn on the subway. She had accepted her sorrow and still managed to find joy and meaning.

As her health wavered and then the Coronavirus brought everything to a stop, she grew older. Like many of her peers, she was hit hard.

"It's okay, we've lived through far worse," she told my brother and me, "we'll get through this."

But the loss of her activities caused her to grow sadder and more disoriented. She didn't take her numerous pills as carefully as she was supposed to and a series of health failures brought her to the edge of death. My mother kept her at home, caring for her around the clock. She knew that at the height of the outbreak, if we took her to the hospital, we'd likely never see her again.

Amazingly, she survived. Don't ask me how—I had already said my goodbyes. She told me she felt such peace near what she thought was the end and that she sensed a presence that assured her everything would be alright. She was ready to go. But she didn't. Instead, she got up and began walking again—with the help of her "old lady stick," as my kids call it.

"Wow," I said, "I thought you would take longer to get back on your feet."

we'll get through this

"I don't have longer," she replied.

"How are you feeling?" I'd ask her.

"I'm feeling," she'd say with a laugh.

The Story of the Goat

There's an old Yiddish proverb Babushka loved to tell me when I was growing up, about a man who struggled in a tiny house with a large family and went to see the rabbi for advice.

"Rabbi, I don't know what to do," he said, "my home is so crowded."

"That's easy," the rabbi answered, "bring home a goat from the farm and come talk to me in a few days."

The man did just that, but he returned even more distraught. "Why did you tell me to bring this animal home, rabbi? It's awful now, I can't even breathe."

"Don't worry," said the clergyman, "bring the goat back to the farm and come talk to me in a few days."

The following week, the man came back. "Oh, rabbi," he said, "my home has become so spacious, so wonderful; thank you."

Do Your Tao

I spent quite a few nights wondering if COVID-19 is the proverbial goat we were forced to bring home. *When we finally overcome it, will we feel delighted to have our lives back to normal?* I'd ask myself. Will we learn to appreciate all the big and the little things more?

What other lessons can we mine here?

I know we are all capable of glimpsing the bright side of life, the silver lining, the calm after the storm. We must either discover this wisdom within ourselves or life circumstances will leave us no other choice (maybe both). Either way, we will all return to the common source of love one day. So, how can we live better now—no matter what's going on—even before or without the solutions?

Life is full of curveballs. We cannot help but feel anguished at times. Still, can we step outside ourselves, outside our turmoil, and contemplate our own return?

However long she lives, Babushka Dina's story, her struggles and triumphs, will inform me the rest of my days. I'm sure you, too, have stories of your own family members or elders who you admire. And if you do not, there is a myriad of impressive historical figures to look at. Keep the strength of our human ancestors close to your heart; it is within you as well. And when you are going through tough times, remember the goat parable.

12

Let Yourself Croak

If you want to become whole, let yourself be broken.
If you want to become straight, let yourself be twisted.
If you want to become full, let yourself be empty.
If you want to be reborn, let yourself die.
If you want to be given everything, give everything up.

The Master espouses one universal formula:
do not be prejudiced by your own views, and you will see,
do not think that you are right, and you will know the truth,
do not boast about your achievements, and you will achieve,
do not be self-contented, and you will grow.
Because in seeking growth you need not struggle or contest
*   with others.*
Only in being lived by the Tao can you be truly yourself.

—TAO TE CHING, VERSE 22

In other words,

Be fluid like the Tao: from broken to whole, from full to empty, and
so on.
Discard your cover-ups and let your spirit shine through.

Surrender

I am ravenous. No longer a food addict, I am hungry for everything else. I want love, life, flesh, and then some.

"The Kisses Store is closed!" my little one squeals in desperation. My cat Regis wriggles his way out of my arms daily.

I desire connection, magic, beauty. To gaze at nature, inhaling—no, *ingesting*—the sweet air. I want deep, soulful interactions—to laugh, conspire with, feel close to friends and strangers, and to know that I matter, and for you to know that you matter. I yearn to be plugged in to the energy of it all.

But, overwhelmed by this hunger, my pattern is to frantically look for shortcuts, for quick avenues to my goals. I drive myself crazy, becoming myopic, walking around with my face glued to my phone screen like so many of us do, constantly refreshing my damn feed. Thankfully, at this point in my life, I have the mind to stop—that's what we need to remember, and often: to stop, to unplug, to come up for air.

I retreat within myself, light a candle, and get quiet. I sit my butt down, close my eyes, and listen.

"If you want to become full, let yourself be empty," I hear. My eyes remain closed until I see only darkness, until I am one with it.

While we cannot expunge the entirety of our human weakness, we can bring ourselves back—from partial to whole, from crooked to straight—like a dance, from human to spirit and back again. *Don't beat yourself up for your basic addictions: scrolling too much, wanting too much, not always being present.* That is what I tell myself as I return inward. I let go of my clenched desires. I give it all up, if only for a moment, and I return to the Tao. *Do what you will with me, Universe,* I invoke.

"Only in being lived by the Tao can you be truly yourself."

I surrender.

Redefine Everything

When I was an innocent Soviet kid, I was obsessed with being good. "I am a good girl, a very good girl," I'd mumble as a toddler. And I was.

For years after coming to America, though, I was in shock. In Riga we all wore uniforms and followed orders. In Brooklyn's inner-city school system, tough kids enjoyed breaking the rules and pushing boundaries. At first I was horrified, then mesmerized, then jealous. Junior high girls talked about blow jobs—I had no clue what that meant. They wore large hoop earrings and dark lipstick; I was not permitted such flamboyance.

By high school, I too transformed myself into a young woman with an edge. I changed my name and adopted an air of mystery. I wore my parents down and purchased cheap makeup. I flirted with sex appeal I knew I possessed but was still very much afraid of. I found friends who bucked the system, and, with them, alcohol, drugs, debauchery. Eventually, I got lost in a persona of my own creation. I knew how to attract males but not how to keep them. I went from disordered eating to love addiction, begging apathetic men to make me whole.

With time, I worked to heal my fragmented self. I shed my pretenses layer by layer (I'm still shedding). I became an open book, revealing my insecurities and humiliations to anyone who cared to listen. I began to connect with everyone I crossed paths with. I owned my confusion, mistakes, and piece-meal identity, and so others recognized themselves in me.

Today, the whole state of the world is in upheaval—this uncertainty is so much bigger than my own identity crisis, I've realized—it's *our* identity crises. Many of us want to toss out the old paradigm but we haven't yet gotten a grasp on the new one. And that's okay. What we can do is start by being honest with ourselves.

Do Your Tao

So let's go there for a moment. Let's ask ourselves, What masks am I wearing in my everyday life? And which ones am I willing to dismantle?

We are often afraid to discard the labels and boxes we find ourselves in because we don't know who we will be without them. But, so what? Let go of the need to know. Choose one area of your existence where you've been hiding behind a construct that isn't really you and commit to letting it go. Perhaps, you always "put your face on" using makeup before leaving the house, or there's an act you tend to adopt when you're around your coworkers or friends.

Instead, if you're broken, be broken; if you're confused, lost, hopeful, eager—whatever it is, let yourself be it without shame. Shed one layer of facade at a time and see what happens.

Who knows how many strata there really are; perhaps they are fully relinquished only once we become air. Still, let us strive to be unabashedly real. When the discomfort passes, we will feel that much more free.

13

Penis on Tippy Toes

Those who stand on tiptoe do not stand firm.
Those who rush ahead do not get very far.
Those who try to outshine others dim their own light.
Those who have power over others can't empower themselves.

When walking the path of the Tao,
this is the very stuff that must be uprooted, thrown out, and left
behind.

—TAO TE CHING, VERSE 24

SO, dear girls (and boys),

See penises on tippy toes for what they are, and for God's sake
don't emulate them.
Be you, do you, worship no one.

A Culture of Dicks

The brilliance and simplicity of "Me too" don't translate well into my birth language. It sounds awkward, more akin to "I also," like something a child might say. On the other hand, there's a phrase a brilliant hairdresser I know coined in Russian that I imagine can work in any language—"a dick on tippy toes" 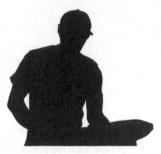 if you want to be crude, "penis on tippy toes" for a more refined description. I often use this expression because it so vividly portrays an endless number of men with egos bigger than their nether regions, which so many of us have had to deal with on our way up, down, or sideways.

"In my great and unmatched wisdom" is something these men might say, as President Trump actually tweeted once. Or they may be a shirtless anchor who puts the moves on you as he critiques your diction (this ridiculous scenario, courtesy of my first out-of-college job)—and a News Director who likes to point out which of your, *ahem*, features looks best on camera. They are men who feel the need to flaunt their possessions, accomplishments, and, most of all power, however meager or grand it may be. But in the most callous of circumstances, they take whatever they want without asking, leaving you feeling used, discarded, broken.

Collateral Damage

Nearly two decades ago I was a college student at NYU's Stern School of Business—with a complete lack of interest in the business world. I dreamed of excitement and creativity, so when I found an internship at a film production company, I was over the moon. It was a revolving door of celebrities and I adored celebrities. *This is amazing*, I thought, escorting Whoopi Goldberg to the bathroom as she told me about peeing in the sink in Catholic School.

I'd been hired by a fun guy in his late twenties. He was relaxed, giving us our assignments and joking around, but mostly leaving us interns alone. When, at the end of the semester, he invited me out for a celebratory drink, I went. I was subservient, naïve, and eager for career advice.

I may have drunk too much for my then one-hundred-pound frame, though I've always suspected there was more in my cup than just alcohol. That night is marred by gaps unlike any I'd ever experienced.

We made our way back to his place so he could show me a movie he was working on. As he ushered me in, I realized his "place" was a single, dark room, with nothing to sit on but a bed, which is where I perched as he put on his film. I wanted to get up then, I wanted to walk away, but I didn't know how. So I stayed.

I vaguely remember being uncased from my pantyhose.

"Why are you crying?" he asked . . . and fade to black.

A few weeks later I ran into a fellow intern, who told me a nearly identical story of her night with our internship supervisor.

"I guess he's got good game on him, doesn't he?" she said.

Oh, that's what that was? I cringed. I felt like the dumbest girl on the planet as hot, sticky shame wove itself into the essence of my being. Only decades later would I even wonder how many reluctant interns followed.

This production house, to which I never returned, ironically made family-friendly movies. Its then-CEO had built his career by working for Bob and Harvey Weinstein, and much of his company's workforce had followed him from Miramax. As #MeToo hit, I couldn't get the company and its men out of my mind. I wondered

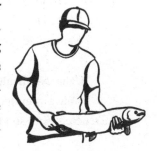

if I'd been yet another fly in the toxic Weinsteinesque net. But, also, I realized a part of the problem was my inability to take up space.

Soviet culture had taught me (and all children) to be demure—legs together, hands in lap, mouth shut. And, as with most immigrant kids, privacy was hard to come by; I didn't have my own room until I was fourteen. By then, I'd accepted the invasion of space that came with being a young developing woman.

I was often in close proximity with other children, which meant being shown penises by older boys and asked to touch them way before I was comfortable doing so—the first time it happened, I was nine. The hands of Russian teenagers were surreptitiously slipped into my shirt or under my butt in packed cars. I learned to dissociate myself from my body, to make myself small and think of Riga.

When the gray-area rape came, I didn't call it that. I stuffed it down with junk, then threw it up and flushed it down the toilet.

My Part

I continued to appease lascivious men as a wannabe on-camera personality. I wore but a bra, thong, and apron in a pilot for Spike TV—a channel aimed at the dumb, young American male. This cooking show was the brainchild of a bunch of food- and women-loving Italians. The exciting part was it had been funded by their famous hometown buddy, who I was surprised to find on set daily. He wasn't intimidating—none of these guys were. So when I ask myself why I paraded around like a half-nude ornament, the answer's pretty simple: I wanted to.

"Want some coke?" the famous actor asked me, "It makes you horny."

"Haha. No thank you," I answered. It was ten in the morning.

"Wait a minute, wait a minute, turn around," his friend then instructed. And so I did, bum bare, a couple cutlets stuffed into my bra. The friend snapped photos on his phone as both men smiled. I felt dirty but significant.

I guess I generally expected men to be idiots—fun, bosom- and butt-loving idiots—I wanted them to like me and to look at me. Just not to rape me.

Now What?

The #MeToo movement may have been a start to disassembling a less than safe reality for women, but it isn't enough. Both sexes still need to go deep within ourselves to dig up the roots of a sexist, racist, homophobic, power-worshiping past. We must constantly check aggrandizement like the Tao suggests, and we must stop bowing down to it at all costs.

"Those who have power over others can't empower themselves." So let's abstain from venerating it, and also from giving it away! Let us all commit to holding onto the might within ourselves and let's teach our youth to do the same—even, even, *even* when it means bucking authority.

I wish I'd admired myself as much as I admired people of influence. I wish I knew that nothing matters more than my inherent magic and that neither accolades nor riches can replace it. My prayer for future generations of girls—and gender-non-conforming youth, and all people for that matter—is a sense of self-empowerment which helps them elicit more respect than I did. I hope they will carry themselves like a loving force to be reckoned with. For, they who stand firmly in their own light will topple tippy-toed dicks left and right.

Do Your Tao

Pretend you are your own daughter, or a niece or a friend's child that you adore. How would you encourage them to carry themselves?

What would you tell them to put up with and what should they always stomp out?

Find that level of love and protectiveness for yourself and imbue yourself with the self-respect and confidence you'd want the aforementioned youngster to have. It's never too late to claim your strength. No matter where you are on your life path, know that you are a worthy, majestic being. Do not seek anyone else's appraisal or approval! Sit up straighter, speak up, and feel your Tao-ness from the moment your feet hit the floor in the morning.

. . . .

it's never too late
to claim your strength

. . . .

14

Alchemy

Something formless and complete in itself was here before Heaven
and Earth.
It is the Mother of the Universe.
For lack of a better name, I call it the Tao.
I call it the greatness of all things, the end of all endings;
I call it that which is beyond the beyond, that to which all things
return.

From the Tao comes all greatness:
it makes Heaven great,
it makes Earth great,
it makes people great.

Thus, to know humanity, understand Earth.
To know Earth, understand Heaven.
To know Heaven understand the Way.
To know the Way, understand the great within yourself.

—TAO TE CHING, VERSE 25

As my little one would yell daily,

"I am Supergirl, I have special powers!"
And she is, and she does; and so do you.

The Greatness Within

Ever flowing, we are constantly returning, the Tao suggests—barreling forward, like it or not. We are all moving toward the same destination; it is our choice whether to do so in grace (though, ultimately, we get back to grace, regardless). En route, greatness is ever present, available to anyone who seeks it, no matter what has happened.

Since humanity mimics the Earth it comes from, like the Earth we experience catastrophic events that alter our landscape forever, and like its elements, we are capable of giving life and wreaking havoc almost simultaneously. But when we step into an astronaut's boots, viewing our little blue dot from a distance, we see only perfection: grooves, colors, elements fitting together to create a magnificent whole. This magnificence—the boundlessness Lao Tzu spoke of— resides within us, just waiting to be unleashed. And while it does not equal a life without hurts, mistakes, or colossal messes, it does grant us alchemy: the ability to turn shit into gold and pain into wisdom.

Think of *kintsugi*: the Japanese art of fixing shattered ceramics by incorporating their brokenness into their beauty. Lacquer is tenderly mixed with powdered gold or silver and used to glue the jagged pieces back together. Every crack becomes a gilded seam.

We too can be like that if we choose—enhanced, rather than diminished by our falls.

Forgiveness

All of us have our trauma, individually and collectively. But these cracks of ours can make us even more special, much like those Japanese bowls.

So, what are the tenets then of living a life of greatness, breaks and all? How do we let in that golden, healing light?

Recovering from trauma is an ongoing process, maybe a lifelong one, but the light can enter quicker if we let it—in rays and trickles, we can begin to feel its warmth, if little by little we accept what is. In that acceptance we surrender to something greater, to the Tao, the Universe, God. We stop fighting everything that's happened to us, and we're finally able to forgive.

Forgiveness, after all, is giving up the hope for a better past.

Like the many women who were sexually violated, I blamed myself most. At first, I blamed myself for not being smarter every time a guy took advantage of me and for liking male attention in the first place. Buying into our society's flawed judgment, I figured since I put effort into looking good and liked getting positive attention, I also deserved the negative—the unwanted, annoying, and, at worst, traumatizing advances and objectification.

Later, I blamed myself for never speaking up, never putting up a fight, for being easy prey, knowing only how to please and to smile sweetly. I faulted the Soviet Union for instilling in me a fear of authority, and my parents who raised polite, amiable children. And also America, whose misogynistic culture I found at every turn as a young girl. I blamed the magazines where women looked like candy and the TV shows that painted us as needy, and the constant appraisal of my looks that came from well-meaning adults when I was growing up. I was a pot of blame and regret, bubbling inside, barely keeping the lid on.

Though I am still working through some of these feelings, mostly, I accept it all—everything I was, everything that happened to me. I am thankful. I am who I am today because of my struggles, not in spite of them. They are what enable me to understand and help others.

As Marcus Aurelius put it, "What stands in the way becomes the way."

And so I forgive the world, my predecessors, my loved ones for their inability to protect me, to protect any of us, really. And I forgive those who hurt me, having learned to devalue girls from somewhere outside themselves. And, like releasing a block of lead, I forgive my human self—for thinking my value lay in my looks and in the eyes of men, for abusing myself with food, for setting impossible standards for my body, for treating myself like a material object, rather than a powerful soul.

Like everyone, I made mistakes. I now try to hold onto the humility of a fuckup and to have empathy for those who are in pain. Some days I succeed, others I fail. Still, I flow forward, recycling my hurt, and bringing value to this world. Even in my base moments, I am returning—we are all always returning to the Tao.

Do Your Tao

Do you know how great you are? A child of the Earth, of Heaven, of greatness itself. Born of the Great Mother, the Divine Feminine, you carry all of her qualities: creation, strength, forgiveness. Your entire life is your artwork—remind yourself of this if you feel stuck in a rut or in a ditch; every moment is another chance to keep painting. Forgive yourself for getting in your own way and forgive whoever else you need to. By carrying anger and resentment, you're only punishing yourself continually. In letting it go, you unburden your spirit to flow on. It is a process of returning to your original completeness— sometimes it's one step forward, two steps back.

For now, think of a single brick of resentment that you're ready to unload. Just one is enough for today. Conjure the situation or person in your mind (or on paper), feel the anger, hurt, loss, and then imagine releasing it—*poof*, back into the ether to disintegrate and come back as a completely different energy. And if its specter ever returns, if you start to feel its heaviness again, remind yourself that you've already let it go and let its phantom vanish as well.

15

Humiliating Love Story

The inner is foundation of the outer,
the still is master of the restless.

Thus the Sage travels all day without leaving her inner treasure.
However splendid the views, she stays serenely in herself.

Why should the lord of a great empire flit about like a fool?
If you abandon yourself to foolishness, you lose touch with your
*   own roots.*
If you lose your serenity, you lose the basis of your own power.

—TAO TE CHING, VERSE 26

And, as any mild love addict must eventually learn,

Do not desert your inner treasure for anyone or anything;
give yourself the very love you're seeking elsewhere.

Playing the Fool

In college, as I ended up drunk in a bed I didn't want to be in, I imploded. I was treading a thin line even beforehand—lacking self-esteem, I frequently sought it in the adulation of others. But after the gray-area rape, my desperateness bordered insanity. I threw myself at the feet of guys I thought could fix me and often got kicked around like dirt. The problem was I had abandoned my inner treasure and forgot about my own power. So when I met Nick, with whom I felt an indelible connection, I lost all command of myself.

This great downfall began like any ordinary romance might—in a cramped massage parlor in Manhattan where, unbeknownst to me, the masseuse pulled back the curtain to show Nick my body splayed out on her table. We were both in our late twenties: I, a chatty actress/waitress renting a squalid room on the Upper East Side, he, a charming stoner who installed audio equipment and lived directly across the street. Almost instantly, I believed we were meant to be.

"I don't fall in love quickly," he warned me in a dark bar one night. "Is that okay?"

"Yeah, sure," I answered, feeling the familiar rush of dopamine.

I did plan to act normal with Nick, I really did. But here's the rub: he was a "serial dater," as his friends called him, and I was a love addict. The minute he began to pull away, I wrote him poetry.

One night, after he dumped me, my girlfriend Carolyn drunkenly threw bagels at his head in a corner bodega, screaming "Leave her alone, just leave her alone." It was like a scene from *All My Children*, which was the soap opera my grandma, mom, and I watched to learn English two decades prior. I penned apologetic soliloquies to Nick afterward and we occasionally hooked up on his cigarette-burnt couch.

He showed palpable interest only once I was ready to skip town.

"Don't forget the best coast," he cooed, referencing my move to California, as he grasped my hand across a candle-lit table—another soap-like clip which kept me up on many a hot LA night.

In Los Angeles where I hoped to become a star, I instead starred in my own fantasies. When my manager dropped me, my bruised little psyche once again turned to Nick. I dreamily envisioned our reunion in New York. Our email exchanges grew more amorous on my part—pages upon pages of *Coldplay* lyrics. Sometime after I threw in the word "love," he stopped answering.

Returning to my parents' home with nothing, I took solace in my cats and my inner world. I got a long-hours, low-paying internship (a thirty-year-old intern in a sea of recent college grads) and moved in with my bagel-throwing protector Carolyn, along with her fiancé. In their spare bedroom filled with golf clubs and Pittsburgh Steelers memorabilia, I bought crystals and devoured self-help books. Still, in moments of weakness, I reached out to Nick, ignoring his silence. He did reply once to tell me he was seeing someone. I wish I could say I never contacted him again, but my obsession petered out slowly, pitifully.

~~Falling~~ *Rising in Love*

As the months passed, I forced myself to stay put, clutching a rose quartz rosary and chanting in Sanskrit. I meditated. I watched TV. I worked on loving my foolish, imperfect self.

One day, logging into my abandoned virtual dating profile, I saw I'd been contacted by a cute, unusually eloquent prospect. I immediately replied to his message. It didn't seem to go through, so I sent him one of those winky faces. Then a "flirt," whatever that meant. The next day, I emailed as witty a note as I could muster. I finally called the site, which confirmed there was an error with my account. After they fixed it, this eloquent prospect named Adam got everything I'd sent him all at once.

"I figured either it was a glitch or you're really into me," he wrote.

I joked it off, embarrassed by my ever-present desperation. Surprisingly, though, this boyish copywriter in sneakers and a hoodie brought plenty of his own turmoil in the form of an almost-ex-wife.

Two weeks after our first date, their official divorce papers arrived while I was lounging in his apartment. Then her mail kept showing up like the ashes of a past life—pamphlets from The New York City Ballet, financial documents, STD test results. Sometimes she called him in tears, though she was the one who had strayed; I pretended not to listen. I was simultaneously jealous and determined to make him mine.

The star-crossed couple's past, filled with separations and hopeful reunions, became my own. I poured over pictures of their backyard wedding and snapshots of them across the globe. Their saga somehow satisfied my need for theatrics—a therapist might have called it transference.

But when I joined Adam on one of his adventures, the chemicals in my brain shifted. *No manmade drama can compete with this*, I realized as my feet touched the silky sand of the Sahara desert. We roamed the streets of Morocco and the Inca trail in Peru. We camped, hiked, and explored until I forgot everything that had consumed me and he forgot his heartbreak. I used to believe he'd saved me. The truth is, we saved each other and we each saved ourselves.

Today, while my full life—and my spirituality—helps keep my restlessness in check, I remain a work in progress. At times, I don't stop myself from looking up Adam's ex or my own former flames. I recently happened upon Nick's wedding photo; it felt like picking an ancient scab—a wound beneath the humiliation. What can I say? I wish he had loved me . . . that I hadn't left a trail of unanswered emails and "accidental" dials in my wake . . . that I hadn't obsessed over him. I wish I hadn't obsessed over anyone.

And, yet, my pathetic past serves its purpose. It is a reminder to tend to my roots daily. To water them and rejoice in them, in all that I have and all that I am—in who I'd actually always been, I just hadn't realized it then.

My empire is vast, my foundation strong. Never again will I go begging for crumbs.

Do Your Tao

When I do find myself groveling for love these days, it's mostly with my children.

"Go away," my little one says matter-of-factly if she catches me hovering over her as she plays. "Mommy, you're ruining my game," the older one proclaims. Even at their young age, they need space and resent feeling smothered. They prompt me to give myself the very attention I seek elsewhere.

Any time you realize you're groveling—in any arena—you too can pivot. Instead, fill yourself up on your interests, on the nature, entertainment, and beauty available to you in this world. Pull back your earnestness and focus on the treasures you already have within you. Then watch what happens.

When I re-align my energy, I get all the hugs, affection, and closeness I can stand, and not just from my kids. As will you. Love flows so much more easily once we stop pleading for it—even if the source is different from what we had expected.

16

Use It

A good traveler has no fixed plans and is not intent on arriving.
A good artist lets his intuition lead him wherever it wants.
A good scientist has freed himself of concepts and keeps his mind
  open to what is.
Thus the Master is available to all people and doesn't reject anyone.
He is ready to use all situations and doesn't waste anything.
This is known as the Tradition of the Light.

The good man is the teacher of the bad.
The bad man is the good man's charge.
Those who do not value their teachers and those who do not take
  good care of their charges,
they are lost, no matter how smart they are.
This is a key point that is often not understood.

—Tao Te Ching, Verse 27

So, remember:

You never know where you will find meaning—
keep your eyes and mind open.
When life throws you a bone, use it,
and when others impress you, use them as an example.

My Zelensky

"Did you know you acted alongside the new president of Ukraine?" my brother texted me when Volodymyr Zelensky was first elected. He included a screenshot of Zelensky's IMDB page.

"Who me?" I wrote back, with the perplexed hands-up emoji overused by every suburban mom.

I read through Zelensky's credits until I found what Alex was talking about: a 2009 Russian comedy called *Love in the Big City* about Russian expats' romantic exploits in New York. I remembered it well.

It was the strangest set I'd ever been on—although they're all strange. While the movie's stars were flown in to film it in The Big Apple, bit parts went to actual expats like me—the one time being foreign helped earn me a paycheck. It was surreal to audition in Russian, to make money in Russian, to play in Russian but as a grownup.

I barely registered Volodymyr back then—the now, world famous Ukrainian leader. He was just a run-of-the-mill actor/comedian starring in his first big film. I'd never even heard of him or any of the other *Rusky* stars in my American bubble. Far more compelling were the loud, nouveau-riche producers, who hung around chain-smoking, drinking champagne, and asking for recommendations on where to shop.

"You could make it, you know," one told me as she poured me some bubbly, "you just need to fix your nose and your chin."

My nose I understood—I knew exactly how Russians felt about Semitic noses (hint: not good)—but my chin?

"What should I do with my chin?" I asked.

"I'd just get rid of the divot."

I never did get rid of the divot; I wasn't actually able to find it. Nor did I change my nose. I didn't quite make it either. But my mom's friend called her from Riga when the movie was released, ecstatic at seeing little Asya on the big screen. So, that's cool, I guess.

Meanwhile, Zelensky parlayed his acting career into becoming the first Jewish president of Ukraine, which used to be one of the most anti-Semitic parts of the Soviet Union. My paternal grandfather's family lived there until the Holocaust; they got out just in time. My father grew up there but moved to Latvia for college, as only a limited amount of Jews were allowed to attend Ukrainian universities.

And yet, here was Zelensky—a Ukrainian Jew in charge, with his sheen of possibility. While everyone else in America was focusing on his role in Trump's impeachment, I was in awe of his seemingly impossible success, not to mention I'd been in a movie with him!

Stepping Stones

When we examine the wayward routes our lives take, in hindsight, they sort of make sense, or at least feed into one another—missed opportunities, chance encounters, ordinary moments that come to mean much more than they seemed to at first. Whether we have concrete plans or not, we can't quite determine where we will net out. And yet, there are miracles and lessons beneath the surface all along, unfolding within the comedy, tragedy, drama of each individual.

Having been on set with Zelensky, I was able to get my first big byline in the *L.A. Times* once he was elected. I realized as I read my brother's text, this was my *in* to the bigger publications I was hoping to crack (other major bylines followed soon after). Then when his name became synonymous with Trump's treachery, I squeezed several more articles out of my connection to the man.

"Enough already," Adam quipped about my overused subject matter, but no matter how much I thought or wrote about it, I didn't grow tired of talking about Zelensky.

I don't know if he will succeed in his efforts to improve his country, especially given how complicated geopolitics are for the former Soviet republic—but I do know he used all situations and didn't waste anything, just like the Tao suggests.

After shooting the movie in New York—*our* movie I should say, having played the vital role of "girl in sportsclub"—Zelensky skyrocketed to national stardom in a comedy series called *Servant of the People*. He portrayed a schoolteacher who became Ukraine's president when his anti-corruption speech went viral. Then, gaining a myriad of supporters, he decided to run for president in real life, similarly promising to fight corruption and usher in change. Using the show's popularity—his party was even named after it: SP, Servant of the People—along with social media, Volodymyr Zelensky was able to beat the incumbent in a landslide. The old-school oligarch was out and he was in; he became the very role he'd played on TV.

His story served as a shining example to me to not waste anything either—to utilize every bad, good, strange experience of my life as a tool for something greater.

Do Your Tao

I used to carry a multitude of regrets about myself and my past. As in, *if I had only been braver from an earlier age, I could have had a head start in my creative pursuits, I could've made it*. But as I grow spiritually, I try not to look back in a judgmental manner any longer—not even on the small stuff: waking up later than needed, forgetting to put something in my daughter's backpack, saying the wrong thing, not saying anything at all. We all are where we are and we are *who* we are—imperfect, idiosyncratic, in process. Is there a way we can use it to our benefit?

Like for me, I am not an early riser, no matter how much I'd like to be—not yet anyway. I never seem to be able to wake up before the kids to do some writing, for instance. But I am a night owl, so I can stay up far past everyone else and do what I need to do. So, there.

If you regularly beat yourself up for your perceived shortcomings or for a decision you had made in the past, try to also reframe your perspective. And when you stress over, say, just missing the subway or not speaking up for yourself (that one's on me, the non-confrontational gal), breathe into the discomfort, then release it, as many times as needed. What happened, happened, there is no point in wasting energy on it other than to retrieve the lessons. Perhaps this mishap will help you do better next time, or maybe you will realize you are good just as you are.

The point is: learn to work *with* yourself, rather than against. And don't dwell in regret.

don't dwell in regret

17

To Want or Not to Want?

The Tao neither contrives to do something nor abstains from
doing anything.
If powerful people would follow it, the whole world would be
transformed—
by itself, in its natural rhythms.
Should a doubt or old desire rise up,
it would be cured by the natural simplicity of the Unnamed.

Freedom from desires is achieved by stilling the mind.
When there is silence, one finds the anchor of the Universe
within himself.

—TAO TE CHING, VERSE 37

Or

Find the stillness beyond wanting, resisting, controlling:
that's where your power resides.

To Want

May I be frank and perhaps not Taoist for a moment? I have a problem with the idea of relinquishing all desire. I simply don't believe *not* wanting is possible in our human form, unless we give our lives over to meditation and quietude in the way of an enlightened Buddhist monk or a selfless nun. For most of us, though, a new desire creeps in as quickly as an old one is satisfied—there's no escaping this cycle, but there *is* power in being aware of it. In fact, there is power in the desire itself.

As the Tao continually teaches us, stepping back from all the striving makes us feel liberated—it's also a big part of actually getting what we want (check out chapter 43 on ManifesTao'tion!). When you realize your wish is not an endpoint but a journey—and not a linear one at that—you're no longer at its mercy; you ride the wave.

It is no wonder, then, that Lao Tzu nudges us in the direction of equanimity—these journeys of ours can be long hauls, and they may require considerable work. But, not to worry: work and struggle are not the same thing; you can enjoy the former. Plus, it becomes less about the chase and more about the unfolding.

We may have wants, but we don't need to suffer in our wanting. And we may control at times, but we don't have to identify ourselves with our controlling. Nor are we the yearning, the resisting, the worrying that colors much of our lives.

So, what are we?

In stillness, we find out; we anchor ourselves in everything and in nothing simultaneously. And from that nothingness—or everythingness—our power emerges. That's when we act, speak, live more effectively.

To Control

I consider myself in charge in one realm and one realm only (for now, anyway): on the home front. And even there, my power is precarious. Mostly, I try to be my young children's shepherd, but sometimes, the lines blur and I become more of a dictator—a benevolent one of course, but a dictator nonetheless. Though, isn't that what parenting needs to be occasionally? It gets confusing.

"You are being so mean to us today," Charlie cried late one night, "*Do this, do that*, you're so bossy!"

I'd been trying to get them to sleep for an hour and it felt like an uphill battle. I had had a long day and experienced that twinge of anxiety, wanting to get them down and get on with my evening. The more they bucked me, the more anxious I got—and so it went, until all three of us were a chaotic entangled mess. At one point I pushed Gigi rather roughly to get her off Charlie who'd already fallen asleep, and I yelled at Charlie to get back into bed after Gigi did inevitably wake her up.

Eventually, my baby fell asleep in my arms amidst her sobs and the older one did too, as I rubbed her tired back. I retreated to my own bed feeling terrible about myself. I *was* mean like I'd been accused. Cue the mom guilt.

Kids are so sensitive to our energy, but we parents throw it around willy-nilly rather than taking charge of it. I know there are many pressures on us, but if we could just center ourselves in the natural rhythms of life and of our children, everything would transform. And yet, we aren't meant to be perfect. It's not possible. We fuck up all the time. I figure as long as we admit our imperfections to our kids and to ourselves, we're okay.

Somewhere between pushing and restraining them, we need to give them opportunities to fall back into their own natural *is*-ness. This takes tremendous patience, as everyone aiming to be a good parent knows. That is why our offspring are some of our greatest teachers.

Do Your Tao

The next time you hurry your kids to get ready, your voice and un-ease rising as you aim to force them out the door, take a pause. Tell them calmly and clearly that they need to leave soon, that otherwise they will be late to _____ (fill in the blank) and step back. Sit or stand with one foot out the door and simply breathe; close your eyes if you need to, and connect yourself to the rhythm of the Universe. Let's see if, given the agency, our children can gather themselves. It may take several tries, but I believe they will surprise us. Plus, if they/we *are* late this time, so what? . . . God, I need this reminder sometimes!

If you don't have children, this same exercise can work in trying to get anyone to do anything—a significant other, an employee, a parent. State your reasoning simply, then back off. This even extends as far as your relationship with the Universe: make clear what you're asking for, then release it.

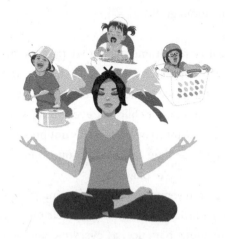

18

The *Egoistka*

The highest good is not to seek to do good but to allow yourself
   to become it—
to give without thinking, without keeping account, without
   seeking gain.
To always adhere to what is virtuous is not true virtue.

When the Tao is lost, we find refuge in the rules of virtue,
When virtue is lost, we find refuge in the rules of kindness,
When kindness is lost, we find refuge in being fair,
When fairness is lost, we find refuge in being gentlemanly.
But if the gentlemanly person is not treated the way he expects,
he pushes away and thrusts aside his counterpart.

—TAO TE CHING, VERSE 38

In other words,

Stop trying so hard to be "good."
You are worthy and good the minute you are born, so just be it.

Swinger of Birches

Have you ever seen trees covered by ice after a freezing rain storm? They look like they're made of heavy crystal, bowed down lower than usual, leaden with the raindrops that were frozen mid-fall. Reveling in this scene one frigid day, I tried to remember if I'd seen anything like it before. I must have—I came from an even colder Soviet winter—and yet, I have no memory of it.

I wonder if my little children will remember their magical crystal backyard, glistening in the moonlight. Probably not.

Perhaps it takes the span of life and disappointments to begin to truly appreciate beauty. Maybe it's our very losses that later force us to stop in our tracks and say, "Ahhh," thanking our lucky stars for being alive to see such magnificence. And, yet, the Earth's gifts lie before us all along, whether we notice them or not. Ever-giving, nature does not take stock of who is paying attention. It doesn't hold grudges when you don't and it never ceases its omnipresent goodness. Its essence is the very virtue the Tao speaks of—water is imbued with it, keeping all of us alive, as is the sun that warms our planet and the trees that help us breathe. Does this kind of purity exist within us as well? It must.

"One could do worse than be a swinger of birches," a barista says to me on this beautiful crystal-tree day, "like Robert Frost wrote."

"The story of my life," he adds and goes on serving me the perfect cup of cappuccino. I look up Frost's poem "Birches" as soon as I leave the coffee shop. Here's a piece of it:

So was I once myself a swinger of birches.
And so I dream of going back to be.
It's when I'm weary of considerations,
And life is too much like a pathless wood
Where your face burns and tickles with the cobwebs
Broken across it, and one eye is weeping

From a twig's having lashed across it open.
I'd like to get away from earth awhile
And then come back to it and begin over.
May no fate willfully misunderstand me
And half grant what I wish and snatch me away
Not to return. Earth's the right place for love:
I don't know where it's likely to go better.
I'd like to go by climbing a birch tree,
And climb black branches up a snow-white trunk
Toward heaven, till the tree could bear no more,
But dipped its top and set me down again.
That would be good both going and coming back.
One could do worse than be a swinger of birches.

The Tao, like great poetry, nudges us towards a more ego-less existence (or a less ego-based one?)—a life in which you don't see yourself as better or worse than any other creature or creation; one where you give without keeping tabs and act according to your own moral compass. What others do, how others act becomes irrelevant, as do outer rules and regulations.

In this way, a virtuous barista is more valuable to the world than an ego-driven president or a profit-hungry CEO can ever be.

Good Girl

Like so many of us females, when I was young I worked very hard at being "good." Polite, obedient, pretty, dainty—that is what the rules, the societies around me classified as good. Being indoctrinated with the strict guideposts of the Soviet Union, I followed them to a T. But the rules that meant you were "good" were not intrinsic to a self-directed child like myself; they were probably not natural to any child. I heard the Russian word *egoistka* a lot, meaning "selfish." As in "don't be an *egoistka*."

My friend recently joked with me that we are both narcissists. I laughed along but felt the discomfort of my past—was I an *egoistka* after all? Being that you're reading a book about me, the answer is probably "Yes," and I'm now embracing it. Because for a long time I was simply confused.

What did it mean to be a good girl, then a good woman? A Soviet girl, then an American woman? A "good mother," a "good wife"—these are all constructs that can drive you mad if you let them. For years, in trying to fit an outward mold, I lost myself.

Thankfully, the gift of time, of aging, is that a woman's internal joy can finally become more significant to her than outer labels. If taking care of my internal self first makes me an *egoistka*, then so be it. For I am the one that shines joy everywhere I go; I am the one who encourages my girls to find their own joy. I am the one who tends to my spirit so that kindness and warmth are only natural— instead of some contrived behavior.

Every day, I grow more comfortable with my authentic being, uncovering yet another layer of magic and potential. Today, even on bad days, off days, bitchy days, I know that I am virtuous at my core. Even when I dwell in the lower vibes of humaneness—I gossip, lose my patience, bicker—I know that I am more than my thoughts and actions, but I still let myself enjoy the full spectrum: the base, gaudy fun and the egoless spirit of serving. I exist in all of it.

Am I encouraging you to be selfish, then? Yes, pretty much.

You gotta fill your tank first. Life is not a show: "Look at me and all of my unselfishness." There are no prizes for martyrs. Give yourself whatever you need to be the whole you; goodness will then flow from you like water. Though goodness, too, can be a work in progress.

Do Your Tao

Giving to others without seeking a reward isn't always easy. We've been primed to think, "What's in it for me?" in this competitive world. A tax write-off?

Even on the smallest scale—when putting a dollar or two in the tip jar—I'd find myself waiting to do it until the server saw me. *Why?* I began asking. *Is it because I want them to feel appreciated or because I want the credit?*

So, I am challenging us to be kind anonymously from time to time. It could be leaving a larger-than-usual amount in that tip jar when no one is looking. Or an anonymous donation on a GoFundMe page. I mean, there are endless possibilities for spreading goodness and I'm sure many of you are doing it already. Next time, pay attention to the inner warmth and freedom that comes with being virtuous without the need for external validation. You can think of it as a selfless *and* selfish study—the observation of the self in the act of giving!

· ·

I exist in all of it

· ·

19

Fly Your Freak Flag

As we learn, we accumulate more and more in the mind;
to tread the Tao, however, we must empty it.
As we empty the mind, we finally lose the sense of contriving.

To win the hearts of all under Heaven, we must always let people be.
If we don't let them be, we will not win their adherence.

—TAO TE CHING, VERSE 48

I'm sure the Queen of Vulnerability, Brené Brown, would agree:

To find belonging—and yourself—you must be real.
So, screw the "shoulds" and embrace the awkwardness.

Being the Idiot

Can I ask you something: How often do you feel like an idiot? Or rather, how hard do you work to avoid feeling like one?

I'd say I find myself there often enough to realize we all do sometimes. And, sure, this is not a comfortable sensation—though by forty, I seem to have gotten accustomed to it. I used to hate it and kick myself afterward, but now feeling like an idiot signifies to me that I'm being my goofy or ebullient or awkward self, even when it's not in line with how others behave. And though shame can pop up when that happens, I've learned to let it pass. Why should I cling to normalcy? Why should you?

Marianne Williamson wrote a passage in her popular book *A Return to Love* that went viral before going viral was a thing (it was published in 1992):

> Our deepest fear is not that we are inadequate. Our deepest fear is that we are powerful beyond measure. It is our light, not our darkness that most frightens us. We ask ourselves, "Who am I to be brilliant, gorgeous, talented, fabulous?" Actually, who are you not to be?

Here's the truth: letting our light shine can be uncomfortable, especially initially. But it's not about trying, it's about removing all the inauthentic layers we've accumulated. Because we've been taught to conform and follow rules and do what other people do— that's been our standard. So in order to break stride, we must unlearn and let go of the rules and the "shoulds." As Jen Pastiloff tells her Instagram community, "Should is an asshole."

Stop it with the "shoulds" and the "that's-what-people-dos." Don't just do what's comfortable to earn your sense of belonging. You belong by being alive, I promise! And if you don't belong, you belong to the non-belongers—to the misfits, the deviants, the outcasts, which can be a helluva good time.

Finding The Misfits

My immigrant childhood made belonging my greatest goal for a while (Adam thinks I'm still too preoccupied with it). I wanted friends so badly when I first got here, but they didn't come easily.

Until one day they did.

By teenage-hood I'd let go of the perfect Soviet girl I had been and while there were still many internal and external hurdles to overcome, my blank slate of a self was ready and open for fun. That is when I found the kind of friends every teen secretly wishes for— accepting, counterculture, reckless. I learned that real belonging has nothing to do with popularity. To this day, I remember that period of being "bad" with utter fondness.

These friends and I were in love with each other. And, admittedly, with cigarettes and pot, and *ecstasy* on the weekends. We huddled together and drank wine coolers and forties well into the night and then reconvened at the diner in the morning.

We wore big, loose pants, and sometimes went to raves in the city, only to reemerge like vampires at dawn, just as the adults in suits headed to work. Somehow, this reality suited me. I still studied after school to keep my grades up, making sure I was responsible before heading out to get wasted.

Through this ragtag social group, I met a beautiful Italian boy named Marco and had the most insane urge to hug him.

"No good," my friend told me, "his ex will never let you have him." Of course, this intrigued me even more. And when we began to date I did in fact have to park my car a block away from his house so that his ex-girlfriend wouldn't slash my tires. But nothing could stand in the way of our magnetic teenage pull.

A year older, and completely disinterested in school, Marco was the opposite of my A-student neurosis. Whenever he was near me, I couldn't take the sensations in my body, until finally, he ripped off a piece of his menthol cigarette pack, wrote his beeper number on it,

DON'T JUST SIT THERE, DO NOTHING

and folded it into my palm. I held it in my hand like a secret treasure, bringing it up to my nose to inhale the *Acqua Di Gio* cologne with which it was infused. It took me days to dial those digits.

As he drove me home after one of our group hangouts, we finally kissed and it was everything a seventeen-year-old outsider had ever dreamed of.

At first, I couldn't believe that cool, beautiful Marco actually found me attractive and lovable. I felt adored. On the one hand, the intensity was too much for my young heart; on the other, it helped me begin liking myself. By finding a sense of belonging with my misfits and then with him, I began to acknowledge the parts of me that were unique and vulnerable—one day I would even embrace them.

Do Your Tao

I am by no means saying that drugs, alcohol, and recklessness are the key to belonging. In fact, it was my ability to straddle two worlds, to remember my sobering goals and responsibilities that kept this period of my life just that—a period, a fun set of memories in my mind, instead of an identity that swallowed me whole. The kids who were unable to move on suffered greatly. What I *am* saying—what the Tao is saying—is to let go of all the shoulds and all the judgments of yourself and of others—to a degree, of course. I for one cannot help but chuckle at those who take themselves too seriously (often, myself included). But, still, to win people's hearts, let them be as they are and let yourself be as you are.

Sometimes you'll be the winner and sometimes you'll be the loser. Who cares? The next time you feel like an idiot, do not go down a shame spiral, but instead, tell yourself, *Good, this means I'm being authentic, rather than some kind of Stepford version of a human.* Witness those awkward moments and let them be.

20

Mystics Wear Leggings

The Master has no fixed mind of her own, she works with the mind
*   of the people.*
If people are good, she is good to them;
if people are not good, she is also good to them.
This is true goodness.

She trusts people who are trustworthy;
she also trusts people who aren't trustworthy.
This is the nature of trust.

The Master's mind is like space.
It is always unsuspecting and innocent like an infant's.

—TAO TE CHING, VERSE 49

So,

Open your mind to the world and you will find teachers
everywhere and in everything—
most incredibly, within yourself.

The Guru Next Door

With eagerness that bordered obsession, I brought a faithful, open heart to my spiritual search—from my very young forays into the self-help aisle, to my studies with channelers, healers, philosophers, psychics. At my lowest point, I was even duped by a gypsy fortune teller in Queens and inappropriately solicited by a bearded Russian mystic in Brooklyn . . . what can I say, every journey has its idiocies.

Finally, after reading all the books and studying with all the teachers (as well as getting certified in Reiki and intuition), I realized it was high time to become my own guru. Following the breadcrumbs, I was simply led back to myself, to my own inner knowing, whether I'm thinking big thoughts or . . .

"Can you braid my hair?"

"Can you sew up my shirt?"

"Where is my computer?" my brood interrupts, as the cat meows indignantly for his food.

Yet, this ordinary, messy life is as empowering as any spiritual practice—in fact, it all works in tandem—there is an unseen order to the chaos.

So when those who are sad, confused, scared seek me out, magically, wise words come out of my mouth or onto the page—which isn't as much about what I am saying as it is about the energy of knowingness I carry within me. This energy allows me to *not* go with the other person into the depth of their despair or their lostness. I remain steadfast.

There's really nothing for any of us to learn, only to remember. So when others forget, I remember for them. I connect to the Tao, I listen to the Universe, I channel Source energy—all of which is simultaneously miraculous and not in the least bit special.

See, anyone who chooses to connect to Spirit is a guru or a messenger of divinity. These gurus are everywhere—at the bookstore, and on Oprah (duh!) but also at a local coffee shop or residing next door. As the saying goes, when the student is ready, the teacher will appear. But when the student is readier, she will recognize the teacher in everyone—especially in herself.

She doesn't cling to her own mind, so the entire world is her mind.

Wise Innocence

The other interesting thing the Tao reveals about a guru or a master is her naïveté, her innocent thinking. Normally, this characteristic is looked upon as weakness, as if there's something lacking. I know I've been told—including by my husband—that I could never be "the boss." I'm "too nice."

"That's not a bad thing," he said, but it felt patronizing. And yet, I'd been patronized so much in my life that I've found a way to use it to my advantage. When you're underestimated, you overdeliver. Plus, I don't want to be the boss, I realized; I'd rather work *with* people, whatever their station in comparison to mine. I'm okay with being soft.

Don't get me wrong, my inability to express what I wanted and what I didn't want cost me a lot in my younger years—sexual encounters I didn't actually desire, other things I didn't want to do but did anyway, cold food I never dared to send back to be reheated. Society can be so unrewarding to the softies, so from time-to-time I'd fight my own essence, and when I did snap, it wasn't pretty. But there must be some kind of middle ground, don't you think?

The Tao Te Ching brings up the process of return so often that I began interpreting its suggestions as ones we usually get to *after* our mistakes and misadventures—the truths we discover (or redis-cover) as we come back to our original nature. Upon dissecting my own path, I realized that, yes, I was born soft, but I always had my own keen sense of fairness within me. At times, life confused me and made me a pleaser; in other instances it hardened me. But through my spiritual growth, I am returning to my original mix of softness and fairness—my own particular innocence.

Here's the deal, friends: If we stay open to all the great minds, miracles, and mysteries around us, we eventually return to the Masterhood from which we came—and while still here on earth, to boot. We can then be a wisened form of innocent: hopeful despite experiences where we've been hurt, trusting despite having been burned, good even to those who seemingly don't deserve it. We cannot do this inauthentically, though—that kind of goodness breeds resentment and martyrdom. Instead, we must try to fill our own tanks in a way that's dependent on no one.

These days, I expect little from anyone or anything in particular, but everything from the Universe. And the Universe always delivers.

Do Your Tao

Who has let you down lately? Your partner? Your "guru"? Your government? Fuck 'em! Not the people I mean, but your expectations. Release them. Right now, with your very next exhale, let these expectations go. One breath for the guy, another for the friend, and on and on and on—including letting go of some heavy demands you put upon yourself—until the only expectation remaining is breath.

Notice how much freer you feel without the weight of expectations and disappointments; if nothing else, your own release is worth it. With this newfound freedom, you can seek and create your own happiness daily. This is also a transformative practice for your relationships—some will strengthen, others simplify or dissolve completely, as the ropes of what is owed loosen. Set your kids free, set your parents free, set yourself free! But as with many an exercise, this one needs to be repeated over and over again.

Let go of the demands in your own mind; work with the mind of the people. Harness a goodness dependent on no one and let it flow to everyone, starting with yourself.

AWARENESS

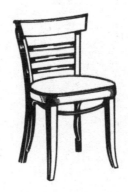

21

What Is Real?

Perfect action, true virtue, supreme power—
this is how the Tao is revealed to those who follow it.

Though formless and intangible, it gives rise to form.
Though dark and unfathomable, it is the spirit, the essence,
    the life-force of all things.

Since before time and space were, the Tao is.
It is beyond is and is not.
How do I know this is true?
I look inside myself and see.

—TAO TE CHING, VERSE 21

Or

There is an energy greater than all form.
Find it for yourself. Play with it.

Questions and Answers

In the 1600s, French philosopher René Descartes famously coined the phrase, "I think, therefore I am." Less famously, he also said, "I doubt, therefore I am." Because it is natural to doubt and to search. But we must be willing to accept an intangible answer, or an unclear one—an answer that changes form depending on who's asking and when.

If we view the Tao as an energy that connects everything, is the source of everything, is within each of us but also everywhere, we can equate it to the Almighty of Western religion. The Judeo-Christian term is God. New age spirituality refers to it as the Universe or Source energy. Whatever we call it, it's been discussed, written about, debated more than we can even fathom. But . . . is it real?

I believe the question *is* the answer. In seeking truth, I try to remain open to every possibility—who am I to say they can't exist simultaneously?

We are all seekers in one form or another: spiritualists, scientists, devotees, atheists—and we all long for love, connection, and meaning. We're basically born with a bold question mark within us. "Why?" the constant demand on the lips of toddlers. "But, why?" they always want to know. It's what we all want to know.

"What is dead, mommy?" and "How does it get dead?"

"How does a baby animal get into its mom's tummy?"

"How did everything get here?" "Why?"

And sometimes, they're the ones with the answers:

"Before me and Gigi were born, we were waiting for you in the sky."

Recognizing Truth

According to researchers, even our long-held beliefs can be questioned. Memories, for one, are unreliable, twisting and turning over time under the influence of other people's descriptions and our own ever-expanding observations. Our brains are complicated machines that interpret the world according to preexisting notions and already-formed neural pathways. That is why two people can perceive the same situation in very different ways.

One man's terrorist is another man's freedom fighter, for example—meaning who the bad guy is depends wholly on who's judging. Our perceptions, surroundings, and teachings form our reality, which differs from person to person.

How, then, can we know what's true?

"I look inside myself and see," wrote Lao Tzu—words which suggest the deepest truths are beyond explanation. They are, at once, personal and universal—think near-death experiences, the feeling of *déjà vu*, or simply witnessing Earth's beauty. These are truths that are larger than *wrong* and *right*.

I know when I hear something profound or am introduced to a grander way of seeing the world, the little hairs on my arms stand on end. I feel moved—intrinsically, intuitively—beyond the mechanical workings of my brain. I feel like I learned something new, yet had known it deep within all along.

Has that ever happened to you?

It is *that* feeling we can rely on for our truth. It is powerful and it gives us radiance, hope, and deep, sourceless joy. This feeling can come from intelligent insights or from the rustling treetops against a blue-gray sky, animals in their remarkable presence, the grass beneath our feet, the smell of the changing seasons, fresh rain, little kids' sweet, sweaty heads, silence.

The truth resides within us and all around us if we are open to it.

Do Your Tao

When's the last time you thought about Truth, with a capital T?

It's worth thinking about, in my opinion.

Somehow, when I ponder "what I know for sure," as Oprah would say, I feel good, I feel hopeful, I feel empowered. So here's *my* Truth, to get the ball rolling:

I know that how I feel within is of the utmost importance—so when it's crappy, I will not be able to create lasting goodness on the outside; I must stop and take care of the inside first.

I also know that an energy we have yet to understand exists and permeates everything. It plays with me when I let it. It will play with anyone who is willing to engage. It's benevolent and I am part of it, so when I'm aligned with this great energy, this Tao, this source of all—well . . . that's when I can do, be, and have anything.

How do I know this to be true? I look inside myself and see. You?

. . . .

?

. . . .

22

Rainbows and Unicorns

The Tao is like water that simmers slowly,
perpetually emitting its energy without boiling over.
It is bottomless, inexhaustible, the origin of all.

With it, the sharp edges become smooth, the twisted knots loosen,
the sun is softened by a cloud, the dust settles into place.

Unfathomable, it is always present,
the common ancestor of all.

—TAO TE CHING, VERSE 4

So, just like the kids did at the start of the pandemic,

Look for rainbows—nurture them and create them.
Because the energy of the Tao is available to us no matter what's
going on.

The Tao of Your Morning Pee

What is this nebulous, esoteric thing that endlessly fills all vessels, that is unknowable yet always present? There go the mind-bending paradoxes again.

I close my eyes and imagine this Tao, which no words can properly describe. I see it as a light, a tingling energy that shines through all things. I feel it as a warmth, a knowing, when I center myself, but also as something deeper than my feelings and fluctuations—present whether I'm reaching for it or not. We can all sense it when we are able to tune into the breath of the world, via nature, meditation, intentional movement, or stillness. But what about all the other times?

It's not an easy feat to get past the daily grind in order to connect with a force that's barely palpable—one which goes beyond physical manifestations. And yet it is our natural pull. When we're hit with uncertainty or loss, we seek solace somewhere outside the struggle of human existence. And even when life is chugging along, there's a quiet but persistent longing for more. Here's the secret though: we *are* more. Always.

We might be people going about our people-ish business. But let's remember, we are also powerful Gods through which the Tao or Universal energy flows, even if we're not aware of it. It is what animates our bodies, as well as the seeds that bloom into flowers. The sky, the hills, the treetops are all an expression of this Tao, which is both mysterious and as common as our morning pee. What I am beginning to understand is that this force is present in every part of our experience—just as much in the mundane as in the extraordinary—in the endless phone calls, spreadsheets, emails, as well as in a house of worship or on a meditation pillow. During sex and bowel movements, and everything in between.

Perhaps we don't need to go beyond our ordinary existence after all, rather, just recall what's already here. Can we feel holy in the most regular moments of our lives, like while washing dishes and cleaning up kids' messes? Can we bless our anxiety along with our joys? It is this ability to see everything as sacred that helps us navigate life's ups and downs.

I remember first reading the Tao Te Ching when I was twenty years old, struggling with bulimia. I was all sharp edges and twisted knots, yearning for a peace I had all but forgotten. There were so many things that happened and didn't happen for me from there to here—a place where I am now grateful many minutes of the day and where I allow myself to go in and out of gloom with the smoothness of a wave. I aim to flow like Lao Tzu suggests; for too many years I bucked the current and suffered. Now, when a sharp edge peeks out in the form of a combatant energy that wants to fight, to resist, I see it, I express it or acknowledge it, and I watch it settle back down. And when I don't, it eventually settles down anyway; it's just a bit louder and clunkier.

So, agitated or stirred up?

Let the dust settle.

Anxious?

Loosen those twisted knots.

There's no need to cling to angst, even when it seems the world or our lives are falling apart. Flowing through the pain, we can choose softness. We can choose to breathe long deep breaths and to search for the Tao within.

Do not hold on to the silly, little resentments of human arguments or wallow in everything that has not gone right. *Settle your dust*, the wind whispers. And when it all seems bleak, look to nature for answers: terrible storms run their course, the sun peeks out again. Sometimes, we even get to catch a rainbow.

The Te of Shit (a.k.a. Storms)

Like many kids, my daughters loved counting and creating paper rainbows which appeared in our neighborhood windows during the first days of the pandemic—little kid drawings to remind us of what's on the other side of the struggle. Because none of us had a choice. We *had* to grow our patience muscle and wait it out.

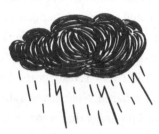

That's the thing with storms: no matter which way one presents itself—whether as an unwanted outer event or the turmoil of our inner lives—we can't force it to pass. Nor can we supress our turbulent emotions. It all needs time and space to dissolve, neither of which is a simple ask. Just being can feel like the greatest challenge in those moments. Still, trying to run from the discomfort precludes us from experiencing the gifts these hardships have to offer. Stay for the gifts!

What's more, as we progress in our spiritual evolution, we *become* the rainbow for others. Obviously, life will never be free of storms, but as we grow, we learn to return to the light that much faster and we hint to others of its existence. Whether with our words, our silent smile, or simply with our iridescent energy, we remind everyone we come in contact with of the rainbow that is on their path as well.

Do Your Tao

I have a confession to make: I believe in everything at least a little bit. During my troubled days of searching (as opposed to my current joyful days of searching), I studied and practiced an energy healing modality called Reiki, also known as the laying of hands. I got to level two out of three in my Reiki training before I moved on to something else, but I had magical experiences in the process. I still practice it whenever the mood strikes me—on a kid or a cat or on my own anxious heart; I lay them hands and remember the rainbow within me.

This internal rainbow we mostly forget about—our chakras— are said to be the energy centers of the human body, with each one having its own vibrational frequency corresponding to a specific color. And they can usually use some attunement.

So whenever you're feeling off or you just want to give yourself some love, remember this tool you now have in your pocket: the laying of hands. Simply picture, feel, imagine energy emanating from your hands and hold them over each of your chakras (see below)— or whichever chakra that's calling out to you right now, and breathe in the healing. This can be as quick or as deep as you want it to be, and you can do it for yourself or for another. Glance at the cursory breakdown below and go for it. If you like it, look into it deeper, but know that just like the Tao, you're always emitting energy. Chakra or Reiki or any sort of energy healing need not be difficult—it's yours to use as you wish, if you wish. If you don't, you can file it under metaphysical info like any of my suggestions and move on. These spiritual tidbits might just come back to you as needed, seemingly out of nowhere, like they do for me . . . which is why I believe in everything at least a little bit.

CHAKRAS

◊ Red is the color of the root chakra at the base of your spine—it's your foundation and stability.

◊ Orange is for the sacral chakra right below the navel—it represents your creative and sexual energy.

◊   Yellow is associated with the solar plexus, which is below your chest—here is your self-esteem and willpower.

◊   Green is your heart chakra (located at your heart, incidentally)—this is your love towards self and others, your relationships.

◊   Blue is your throat chakra at the center of your neck—it corresponds to communication and self-expression.

◊   Purple (or deep indigo) is at your third eye, right between the eyebrows—it represents intuition.

◊   White (or purplish white) corresponds to your crown chakra at the very top of your head—this is your higher consciousness and spiritual connection.

23

How *Not* to Fear Emptiness

Thirty spokes join together to make a wheel,
but it is the center hole that allows the wheel to function.
Clay is molded into a pot,
but it is the emptiness inside that holds whatever we want.
Wood is fashioned for a house,
but it is the inner space that makes it livable.

The usefulness of what is depends on what is not.

—Tao Te Ching, Verse 11

Thus,

Do not rush to fill the void inside you.
Acknowledge it, honor it, use it.

Embracing the Void

Who in this world is truly comfortable with non-being? It sounds a little bit like dying, right? Yet when we drench ourselves in all being all the time, we get tangled up into a frenzy. This hit me over the head when I misplaced my wallet, both my daughters' shoes, and my car (yes, that big chunk of metal on wheels) in the same day. A version of the kind of mishap that happens to all of us from time to time, but how often do we stop to ask ourselves why?

Ultimately, the tornado subsided. I found my wallet, car, the wee shoes. Everything seemed to return to its rightful place once I began to organize my haphazard thoughts and undertakings—once I was forced to pause.

We may work with being, but non-being is what we use, Lao Tzu reminds us—like the space between the walls in which we live, and the emptiness inside a vessel that is ours to fill. There is a void within us as well, one that frightens many of us as we try to cram it with the aforementioned addictions, or the endless plans and activities which make us feel oh, so important. We try to stuff this void with love, which works for an instant—only as long as we are infatuated, smitten, head-over-heels. We attempt to plug it with children, who pull away from us before long, needing to live their own lives, make their own way.

But what the Tao Te Ching is telling us is to *use* the void, instead of simply filling it, to embrace it. I mean, why are we so afraid of this nothingness from which everything emerges?

While it is true that action is needed to make things happen, action itself is not enough. That which is *not* is the birthplace of our dreams. It is what spurs us to find love, joy, fulfillment in the first place.

I was on the dating circuit for many years, like tons of other twenty-something women wanting the best for themselves. Sometimes it was fun; often, it grew tiresome. "I was worried about you," my *babushka* told me. I'm not sure her generation approved of the *Sex and the City* lifestyle. Though mine was more like Sex and the City and Tears in the Suburbs, where I lived with my parents.

My dating life was robust but cringe-worthy. I got entangled with men I obsessed over but who were barely interested in me. I spent time with those that didn't get me and probably never could. Yet, with each less-than-great experience, I learned about myself and my needs. Without realizing it, what I didn't get, what didn't happen, was as necessary as what did.

Eventually, I took the time to reflect on my experiences and to get clear about what I wanted to create. I sat in silence many an evening, reaching a state of nothingness. From that state I imagined the kind of relationship I wanted to experience. I chanted and held crystals and lit candles, because I'm into that kind of thing. And as I quieted my mind, I felt connected to a power greater than the physical. Then, I took the action of going online, *again*. This time, I met my partner immediately, albeit awkwardly.

"I manifested you out of thin air," I like to joke with him. Because I kind of did—from non-being he be'd his a$$ into my life.

Flowing

To access a sort of magical non-being state, we need to stop our incessant doing—or become the doing so completely that the action itself falls away.

Meditating is a good option. For inconsistent types—you know, the kind that fall asleep while trying to meditate (*who, me?*)—well, even a little is better than not at all. I don't believe in all or nothing anymore. A bit of this, a bit of that: the deepest inhale, a poem, a walk, a song . . . getting into the flow state. I do whatever works for me, what helps me disconnect from the madness. None of this is set in stone.

So, find something that fits who *you* are—something that gets you "in the zone," as they call it —i.e., flow.

This is the terrain of masters like Michael Jordan and Mozart, as well as climbers like Alex Honnold. The 2018 documentary *Free Solo* portrays how he climbed El Capitan, a three-thousand-foot granite wall in Yosemite National Park, by utilizing flow. He accomplished his climb without rope or safety equipment—which is nuts, let's be honest—after years of preparation and planning. Ultimately, though, he had to enter the flow state, using the very non-being referred to in the Tao Te Ching.

Mihaly Csíkszentmihályi, a Hungarian-American psychologist who authored *Flow: The Psychology of Optimal Experience,* was the first to actually identify the concept—a state where you're so immersed in what you are doing that you lose yourself in the activity completely, letting go of your sense of self. Here are its characteristics:

1. Intense focus on the task

2. Clarity of goals and immediate feedback

3. The activity is intrinsically rewarding

4. Action and awareness are merged, bannishing self-consciousness

5. A feeling of effortlessness and ease

6. A sense of control over what you're doing

7. A distorted perception of time

8. A balance between challenge and skills

Csíkszentmihályi believes you are happiest when you enter this zone. Alas, you cannot stay there indefinitely—you'd forget to eat, sleep, and tend to other parts of your life. That is why both the spokes and the hole in the center are needed to move the wheel; both the being and the non-being make up a balanced life.

Do Your Tao

I'm pretty sure we all experience flow in our lifetimes; we just may not be conscious of it at the time. Sex, when it is good, takes place in that state, as does a captivating conversation—or anything else you enjoy enough to swallow you whole for a bit. Look over the elements pinpointed by Csíkszentmihályi and pick something to get you there. Maybe try a totally new endeavor—you'd be surprised how encompassing novel activities can be.

As someone who thought she was afraid of heights, I was shocked at how much I liked climbing. Charlie fell in love with it at an indoor climbing gym and began dragging us there regularly. I got a little better every time—and to my astonishment—I got in the flow while doing it. It's not something I do that often, and it will probably never be a big part of my life. Nonetheless, I love the way it brings my mind sharply into the present moment: the next ledge to grab onto, the next footing to locate, to pull, to grit, to float. I get it, Alex Honnold, I get it!

Such activities peppered into our lives can do a lot for us. So, find something, anything—it doesn't have to be big—to drink in a sip of flow.

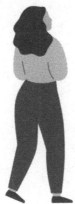

24

Irrational Woman

Express yourself completely, then keep quiet.
Be like the forces of nature:
when the gale blows, there is only wind,
when a downpour comes, there is only rain.
The wind and the rain are from Heaven and Earth and even these
*   do not last long.*

If you open yourself to the Tao, the Tao will eagerly welcome you.
If you open yourself to insight, you are at one with it and can use it
*   completely.*
If you open yourself to loss, the lost are glad to see you.

Open yourself to the Tao and trust your natural responses—
then everything will fall into place.

—TAO TE CHING, VERSE 23

Or

Feel fully.
Then let it all go.

Repression/Expression

Have you ever seen a little kid get mad? It's glorious, really. Their rapid mood swings, which are totally normal developmentally, result in a child-sized soap opera. It's quite a show.

"Gigi Sweetie" can charge like a wild beast, for example. She'll throw something across the room so hard, you better duck, and fast. Charlie is mellowing out as she grows, but still, when she's truly upset, the downpour is intense; I have a feeling it always will be, and that's okay. It takes a minute for her to explode, another minute to gather herself, and then she's back, deflated, often crying, but whole.

I fight like that too sometimes—I have no doubt where they get it from. It's "childish" I've heard, or "crazy." "I can't unsee that," Adam once said after I blew up at him. I'd been all wind. Or all rain or something.

The thing is, repression equals eventual explosion. And, often, we don't even realize what we're repressing until we do explode. Is it ideal? No. Is it alright? *I* think so. We are all doing the best we can with our limited vantage point. My hope is that by allowing our kids the freedom of emotions, they will better understand what's going on inside them. Maybe we will, too.

What I have learned about myself thus far, as just another flawed human, is that I can be too sensitive and too easily offended or hurt. I take the air out of my anger without outbursts whenever possible—I remember the Tao, opening myself up to insight, letting the clouds pass. But at times, much like a kid, my emotions get the better of me and I blow up. It doesn't last long. And after the storm, the sun follows.

I am no longer ashamed of these episodes (well, maybe just a tad). If you're anything like me, I invite you to also let go of your self-judgment and to replace it with awareness.

By observing ourselves, we grow. We are better able to transform our raw reactions, becoming less gale and more breeze. But first we must stop constantly repressing them.

We, women, get a bad rep for being emotional creatures—Hollywood romcoms are filled with irrational leading ladies and confused men unsure of how to handle them. In the workplace, we strive to contain ourselves for fear we will be judged according to these female stereotypes. However, within each of us, just like within the Tao, there are feminine and masculine energies, and neither gender has ownership over feeling deeply.

We all deserve to express our feelings, as many moms of boys are currently teaching their sons. It's time to stop fearing the fluctuations within us. Emotions, like weather, are part of existence. Even when they get out of hand, they are only a smidgen of who we are—beings that are far wider and broader than our hurts and grievances. Can we feel them and also observe them from a higher perspective, being small and great simultaneously? And then, can we let them go?

We can.

The Luxury of Presence

I love those moments in life that take me out of my funhouse of a mind, out of myself in a sense—away from all the sensitivity and overanalysis. That is why I enjoyed acting and why I threw myself into painting and drawing as a kid. It's why traveling, especially the adventurous kind, feels like a break for the brain, as do experiences of flow.

But when we are busy adulting and keeping up with our chaotic world, these other-worldly instances are fewer than we'd like. So what is the antidote?

The solution, once again, is presence. After all, the reason a state of flow is so appealing is because it takes us out of our problems and concerns, our daily grind, and lands us smack in the middle of the present moment. However, glimpses of this mindfulness can be incorporated into our everyday lives, as we wash dishes, tend to the children, or run from one meeting to another.

"Open yourself to the Tao, then trust your natural responses," said Lao Tzu—an opportunity which exists in the space between stimulus and response. If we can tap into that moment, if we can enter that space, our response will come from our higher selves (versus our base selves). It will allow us to move from mindlessness to mindfulness.

By being less reactive, we get to remain in the peace and joy we've been cultivating. I mean, we'll inevitably get knocked out of it, but that's why we arm ourselves with practices which get us back to equanimity as swiftly as possible.

Remember: nothing matters more than how you feel. Nothing.

Do Your Tao

Many of my mornings begin with kids jarring me awake. As soon as I can, though, I steal a few minutes for myself, whatever point in the day that is. Sometimes, all I have time for is a couple mindful breaths; other times, a morning meditation or a spiritual recording. But lately, I've realized that just driving my car in silence after drop-off can be enough. I look at the trees, the sun or rain or snow. I smell the smells.

It takes just an instant to reconnect to the greater energy of the Universe. It's not about the amount of time or effort but the depth of that connection. If you simply look up when you exit your front door in the morning—look up and see the magnitude of existence—that is enough. Commit to that remembrance, to allowing yourself the luxury of being present whenever possible, and feel the magic!

25

We Are All One

Hold your male side with your female side,
hold your bright side with your dull side,
hold your high side with your low side—
then you will be able to hold the whole world.

When opposing forces unite, the Tao inside you strengthens.
Flowing through everything, it returns you to your eternal
*   beginning,*
and you become as a little child.
If you embrace the world as it is, it returns you to the Uncarved
*   Block.*

When a block of wood is carved into utensils,
the Master uses them yet keeps to the block because of its limitless
*   possibilities.*
Great works do not involve discarding substance.

—TAO TE CHING, VERSE 28

Thus,

Honor the opposites within you:
feminine/masculine, hard/soft, introvert/extrovert.
Allow for diversity within and then rejoice in it without.

Girls Will Be Boys

We live in a time when many of us are realizing that the limited categories into which we separate people are simply insufficient—gender and sexual orientation, for instance, are not at all as clearcut as straight or gay, male or female. But not everyone is ready to accept this. Perhaps people who viewed the world a certain way their entire lives feel threatened by the more nuanced reality; maybe they're afraid of the nuances within themselves.

Still, our spiritual evolution, our awakening naturally leads to the breakdown of labels and boxes, the ushering in of unity, both internally and externally.

The world cannot be considered evolved when your race, gender, and the religion and country you're born to dictate so much of your life and your opportunities. And so we move forward little by little—by truly getting that no one category of people is better than another, by facing our indoctrinated ways of being, and by realizing that both sexes exist in each of us.

Looking at identity from the perspective of the Tao Te Ching, the need to label yourself as anything at all seems unnecessary.

As the mother of two girls, I've discovered their genders have little to do with who they are as humans, no matter how many times people tell me, "well . . . boys are different."

"I love my two sons," Adam says when they wrestle for hours, mercilessly and with insane vigor. They are also fearless climbers, scaring the crap out of me at times. They're physical and boisterous, and girlish too—as are many a boy!

I guess I knew this on some level, which is why when Charlie was born, I refused to buy her anything pink. I mean other people gifted all the girly accoutrements, but I adamantly stuck to clothing I thought was cool and gender-neutral, or at least not as prescriptive. Well, the joke was on me. For several years, my firstborn refused to

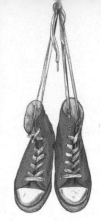

wear pants. Ever. She was all dresses all the time. And skirts, tutus—a frilly, sparkly, unicorn-and-rainbows-covered fairy-tale, her luxurious, golden curls cascading down her back. At the same time, she balked at being called pretty or a princess or any other description that felt imposing to her.

"I'm just Charlie Mirabel Kanzer," she'd state gruffly.

Then one day, *poof* went the dresses, replaced with sneakers and calluses on her hands, due to all that monkey-barring. She taught me to stop labeling her and she did so without words, simply by being her "feminine" and "masculine" self. And little Gigi has always embodied that unity. As a toddler, she raced her toy cars and cuddled her baby dolls simultaneously. She is equally tough and sweet, a strong powerhouse and a nurturer.

If we look to our children, they will show us they are both soft and indomitable, boyish and girlish, and that they are ever-flowing, ever-changing.

It saddens me that previous generations were raised to strictly adhere to gender norms. I didn't have toy cars, for example, and neither did my girlfriends. I never saw little boys pushing cute strollers with dolls in a way that they do today, at least here in New York.

I believe if we give kids the freedom to explore everything, they will net out where their inherent nature leads them—rather than being who society tells them they should be: dainty little girls or macho boys. Their authenticity, not their gender, is what matters.

The Great Unity

Growing up, I felt the world seemed incredibly dualistic—there were very clear demarcations of shoulds and should-nots, desirable and undesirable. Internalizing this duality, I collapsed under the weight of my own mind and have been searching for Great Unity ever since.

Sometimes it proves elusive, other times everything within me and outside of me falls into place. I don't quite know yet how to manifest this unity consistently, but I can tell when I am there, aligned with the Tao. I recognize it because it feels like ease, even as I am bone-tired. It feels like insuppressible joy, even as I face uncertainty and change and melancholy. It feels like clarity, belief in myself, my abilities, and my purpose. Within me, this Great Unity is a keen sense of goodness and humor. It lies beneath all the human drama of my own life, not to mention the baggage of my ancestors—the pain and bewilderment of my mother, grandmother, great-grandmother, passed on through the umbilical cord. Beneath this turmoil is pure light.

When we learn to simultaneously balance the hard and the soft within us, we find peace. If we accept every forceful and gentle feeling, every noble and selfish desire, we can be whole. We can be unapologetically male, while holding onto our femininity. Easy? No. Still, we can do it.

Do Your Tao

Think about aspects of yourself that are male and the ones that are female. Which are you comfortable with and which do you suppress?

Here, I'll go first as an example:

A facet of my femininity that I love is my effortless nurturing of children and animals. The masculine quality within me that I'm less than comfortable with is my competitiveness and drive. I get jealous when I see people achieving the kinds of things I want to achieve—and I immediately feel uncomfortable with my jealously. But "jealousy" is just a label that we give each other when we want more and feel it intensely. What I'm working on now is transforming this jealousy into fuel. When I feel it, I take it as a signal to myself that perhaps that's the direction I want to go in. I stop judging it, I bless those who inspire it; then only fuel remains—one that's neither feminine, nor masculine, but unified.

26

Society's Car Crash

Putting a value on status will create contentiousness.
Showing off possessions will disturb people's daily lives.

The Sage governs by emptying people's minds and filling their cores,
by weakening their ambitions and strengthening their resolve.

Practice not doing . . .
When action is pure and selfless, everything will fall into place.

—TAO TE CHING, VERSE 3

In self-governance,

Beware of the imagined judges for whom you can end up
performing your life away.
You need neither be an influencer, nor a puppet—
You are Spirit. Own it.

Just ~~Do~~ Don't It

In his guide to the Tao Te Ching, *Change Your Thoughts, Change Your Life,* Wayne Dyer wrote that he interprets any mention of governance in the text as more than simply political advice and looks at how it applies to our interpersonal lives and to those we care for. I'd go even further to view it as counsel on how to govern *ourselves* and our inner worlds (along with, you know, a city or a queendom, if that's your jam). What I wonder is, can we can take charge of our minds by emptying them, at least occasionally, as Lao Tzu suggests? By weakening our own hungry ambitions?

This might have seemed like a tall order in yesterday's "Just Do It" culture, but it feels possible now, necessary, even.

Ambition doesn't have to be king; work doesn't have to demand endless devotion. Our society had put too much value on achievement, too much emphasis on doing, and not enough on being—so when the world came crashing to a halt, despair ensued. At the same time, a light was shined on this deep imbalance that limits authentic happiness—a lesson I too learned the hard way . . .

As a bookish Soviet girl, I studied hard and harder. While I loved to paint, sculpt, write poetry, I felt the pressure to be practical. No matter what, through all of my trauma and drama, I got straight A's. And, I can't help it, I'm still proud of them; everyone had always been so proud of my A's. They equaled success, a promise of money, value, status.

"Let's see what kind of jobs are listed most often in the paper," papa counseled me when I was deciding on a major.

"Hmm," he pulled open the *Sunday Times,* "finance, finance, business something-or-other, marketing, finance."

I picked Marketing because it sounded vaguely interesting. But by the time I transferred to New York University's sleek, austere Stern School of Business, I was in trouble. What I mean is my sanity was in trouble, not my grades—God, no! I graduated *summa cum laude* a few years later. Internally, though, I was imploding. I don't think there was anyone in Stern who cared less about production bottlenecks and accounting principles than I did. Or that Lehman Brothers and Goldman Sachs were coming to campus. The anxiety beating in my chest screamed, "Escape *now*" and I usually did, stuffing my face in Penn Station and purging my worries and donuts in my family home on Long Island.

I graduated a semester early and, as if by design, got into a massive car crash a few days later. Some woman ran a red light and smashed her wheels straight into the middle of my ennui, leaving me unconscious and sliced up near the eye—which all in all is better than in the eye. I'm not exactly sure what happened to my brain that day, other than a concussion, but I was at peace for the first time in ages. I felt like I got a reprieve from life—and, truth be told, some potent Percocet.

"Rest," the doctor said, "lots of rest."

I rested.

My run-in with the fragility of life made me realize that a career in business was impossible for me. I can't even picture what that would have looked like. Instead, I decided I needed to be on television. I *had to* be. I wanted to prove to my immigrant community that there were other fields besides business, law, and medicine—and to show my American bullies how wrong they were about me. I wanted to show myself. Plus, it felt good to have a mission. It still does.

After an intensive course in news, I got a barely-paid gig as a local writer and teleprompter-operator. I shadowed reporters every chance I got and made mountains of clunky VHS tapes to send to news directors. I was dedicated. I *was* my ambition. But when I landed my first on-air job, the high dissipated all too quickly. With every assignment, every live shot, I was less and less enthusiastic. I felt trapped in a role I'd worked my butt off to get; only later did I realize how common of a predicament that is.

Most of us have been taught to believe good things don't come easily, that we must work as hard as necessary to get what we want. If it feels like an uphill battle, we push even harder. Through sweat and sheer will we drown out the voice within us—the one that is aligned with Source, with God, with the Tao.

When I finally admitted to myself how dissatisfied I was, I returned to square one. *What am I supposed to do in the world?* I asked over and over again. I had other roads, other goals, some fruitful, some not. But over the years, I learned to listen to life itself instead of clenching my fists and plowing ahead. I let meaning come to me, rather than capturing it like a hunter and wrestling it to the ground.

I see the Coronavirus as our society's car crash (or a goat, I guess). Even as the effects of the pandemic were far-reaching and devastating, we were invited to accept the gift with the curse and allow our ambition to take a breather.

We were invited to embrace stillness, to deemphasize our endless plans and aspirations, to strengthen our connection to the Universe, and to practice not doing. It was, and always is, a good time to ask for guidance from something greater than our human selves.

"Use me, God, use me" is Oprah Winfrey's constant prayer. And look where it has gotten her.

If you take a pause to align yourself with Source, your ambitions will not feel like ambitions, they will feel like purpose. You will start doing what you know you are supposed to be doing. The struggle will lessen. You will feel at peace both with yourself and with the world at large—not all of the time, of course, but enough of the time.

Stop the Thumb

Speaking of the world at large, who knew we'd be able to reach it from our beds? (Maybe futurists did.) Who knew we'd be reaching for it so often?

Too often.

Long before Facebook and Instagram, the Tao suggested we *not* focus on displaying what is desirable. But we do more than just display it now—we are obsessed with it, constantly primping ourselves for our virtual audience, who in turn are primping themselves for us. Yet, while social media brought our performative needs to the surface, it did not create them.

 Maybe this trend started at the height of Mad-Men-style advertising, when we were taught to judge a woman's value—and that of her man—by the size of her diamond ring. Or maybe it always existed in the fiber of our human bodies. Either way, we are now able to produce the most grandiose reflections of our base selves on platforms that profit from our insecurities. Don't get me wrong, these platforms that swallow hours of our lives have also served as a force for good, disseminating vital information, reconnecting lost friends and family members. But something as powerful as the Internet requires an extra dose of mindfulness that, frankly, we were not prepared for. Most of us cannot help ourselves from getting sucked into the social media fray, contributing with our own bombastic posts (myself included).

"Look at me, *look at me*," we all beg.

"Look at my happy family, our grand vacation, my new shoes, my engagement ring," our ego sings. Even in the midst of quarantine, we had to post our color-coded calendars, our sourdough starters, and our impressive projects with the kids. Me—I had few projects in the works other than taking them into the woods and frolicking, and I often questioned myself when I saw other parents' exploding volcanos or baking extravaganzas. My ego felt lesser than.

"The ego is your self-image, it is your social mask, it is the role you are playing. Your social mask thrives on approval," said Deepak

Chopra in *The Seven Spiritual Laws of Success*. But can it ever really get enough likes, hearts, and emojis to satisfy its needs?

Our constant displays make us feel good but for a moment. "Look at what I have," we seem to be saying, waiting for the thumbsups to pour in. What we don't see amidst the likes and comments are the people now thinking, "Look at what I don't have."

And yet, this ever-present bulletin board is a concrete part of reality now, as is our need to check it and to add to it—so is there a way to interact with it mindfully?

As I got bolder with my writing, I drew more attention from people who don't know me, and initially, I'd find myself in many an Internet wormhole. I'd pour over the mixed reviews to my articles, but I would focus most intently on the negative ones:

"Lame," "horrible woman," "control your children."

Cringing at the vitriolic comments, I kept checking for and reading them anyway—until, finally, I realized that's an egoist trick as well. Just like a naughty toddler, the ego drinks up negative attention as much as the accolades. It's the attention it's after—the positive kind puffs it up, the negative confirms its greatest fear of inadequacy, and round and round we go—a heightened emotional state making us feel alive. But let's stop and ask ourselves, do we actually want to be a walking tabloid? Or a glossy perfectionist magazine? Or a cautionary tale? And do we really want to allow the media to control our state of being?

Along with giving us an outlet for exhibitionism, the Internet holds us captive with dramatic headlines, continuing that heightened state our egos are after. So, finally, we are no different from alcoholics going to bed with bourbon—read: smartphones—at our bedside table. Unless we take charge of our addictive tendencies, they will eat us alive.

Do Your Tao

First, if we're going to share our lives with friends and strangers, let us at least be honest; let us show our vulnerability, our fallacy, our tattered lessons as often as we share our admirable facade—more often would be preferable. That way our exhibitionism can morph into truth and truth can foster connection.

Second suggestion: every other time you reach for your phone for no apparent reason, pull your hand back. I'm kidding with the "every other time" bit—I'm not the boss of you. But do be mindful of your own proclivities, which seem to be nearly universal. If your scrolling thumb tends to act of its own accord, as mine does, fold it back into your palm occasionally and do something else. It'll be fun, I promise—not a punishment, but rather a shift. Watching something funny or soothing or even mindless on TV is more beneficial than another hour of social media addiction (but *just* TV, not TV *and* scrolling, you multi-tasker). Not to mention, you can always, like, I dunno, read a book?

Whichever way works for you, be the kingpin of the Internet and not vice versa. You be the boss!

27

The Art of Manipulation (or Is It Perception?)

The best leaders are those the people hardly know exist.
Next come those who are loved and praised.
Then come the ones that are feared;
the worst are those that are despised.

If you don't trust the people, they will become untrustworthy.
If you don't trust yourself, how can you trust anyone else?

The great ruler speaks little and his words are priceless.
When what needs done gets done, people will say
  "How natural and easy it is!"

—TAO TE CHING, VERSE 17

So,

Choose to trust others, starting with yourself,
and allow everyone a sense of agency.

Ruling Yourself

Trusting ourselves is a power many of us—especially women—relinquished for centuries. God knows, I still have room for improvement. It used to take me ages to choose what to eat at a restaurant, for instance, and I inevitably wished I'd ordered what someone else had on their plate.

"You're not very good at making decisions," my husband said once, nonchalantly. His comment stung. *I should be good at making decisions*, I thought. I'm a smart, capable gal, fully aware of the paradox of choice and its limitations. So, why would I delegate so much of the decision-making in our relationship to him?

I've realized that my *not* making decisions is also a choice. I can be overly emotional, while Adam is highly logical. I am lazier than him when it comes to research and documentation (he has spreadsheets and lists for *everything*). Mainly, he is confident in himself and his abilities, whereas I tend to flail about, not trusting myself to decide . . . or, rather, I used to.

I wouldn't make the hard calls because I was so afraid to be wrong. In this way, I was often stagnant. I spent my twenties unsure of which career to choose; thus I didn't get far in any. When I finally went big and moved to Los Angeles to pursue acting, it took less than a year for me to realize that decision was wrong, though I prefer to look at it as a necessary detour.

Here's the thing: in making choices, we may take some erroneous turns and we may fail, but that is as much a learning opportunity as anything else. When we realize that failures and mistakes are simply stepping stones, moving forward becomes easier, and we can trust the journey.

. . . .

failures are simply stepping stones

. . . .

Ruling Others

Since children often push the very buttons we need pushed, my fear of making decisions came up immediately. I mean, think of everything you need to decide before the child is even born: their name, their birthplace, what they will wear, ride, and sleep in. Then, as I was the one who spent the bulk of the day with our babies, it was on me to act on their behalf—initially, a paralyzing task—I could barely choose for myself, how was I supposed to do it for a whole other, then two other human beings?

With experience, though, I have freed myself from the gargantuan weight of making the correct choice. Our kids' activities, schools, camps, even the foods they eat, are not as significant as we make them out to be. These are all opportunities for them to learn and to grow and to make mistakes—as well as to watch their parents make mistakes. Nothing is as vital as we think it is, except for an open heart and communication. In a way, the pandemic highlighted this truth: that our children are more resilient and flexible than we could imagine, that even without all the fixings we spend so much time picking out for them, they recalibrate and have fun. They may act out while processing change, but they find their flow—usually faster than we do. And the process equips them for life better than any class or activity we stress over.

The more all of us figure out this flow thing and the more we are able to be in tune with the Tao, the easier it is to trust ourselves and to trust the bigger picture—and in the light of trust, the fear of darkness subsides.

Becoming the Great Ruler

As you read these words of mine, there's something I must admit—I talk a lot—that is why I am able to write them. I mean, I talk too much, some may say. Many a night, Adam falls asleep while I am still talking. Every paramour I ever had joked about how much I talked. It is a part of me that's hard to integrate with many a spiritual teaching, but I have accepted it nonetheless. And I've met many women (and some men) who love to converse as much as I do. So, you know what? I'm no longer sorry for being a Chatty Cathy; I'm pretty sure it's my *Te*, my nature. Anyway, it's the intention behind our words that matters.

If you're like me, *Hiiii, let's chat!* And if you're not, let me explain. I use my many words to understand the world, as well as to connect with others. My ability to communicate means no one in my presence will be left feeling uncomfortable or alone. I may talk and talk, but my parables and questions invite others in.

So when I read "The great ruler speaks little and his words are priceless," I believe the Tao is referring to a different kind of speaking than the convo-therapy my chatty pals and I engage in. We're not "rulers" after all. Instead, it's pointing at the proclamations that anyone in a position of power and leadership makes, which can be excessive and obnoxious—think a micromanaging boss or an over-tweeting politician.

The Taoist way of ruling calls for putting a lot of trust in those you are in charge of, so when you do instruct them, that trust is reciprocated—your words are "priceless." The Master, by mirroring his people, makes them feel in control—as does a masterful parent.

Before children can even speak, they yearn for independence—they yearn for Tao-ish parenting and for a sense of agency. Gigi can take this to the extreme, wanting to rule the entire family herself. But all kids like to feel capable.

"Do you need help?" I'd ask Charlie when she was a toddler.

"I like to help me myself," she'd reply.

And when I was still getting used to the whole mom thing, her preschool teacher told me that to avoid fights, we should put only seasonally appropriate clothing within her reach—then she still gets to make her own choice while we know she will not freeze. Makes sense, right?

Kids are actually pretty easy to direct with choices—or "deals" as we call them: "Do you want to leave now so you have time to watch TV before bed, or stay longer and no TV?" We also often succumb to bribery and empty threats—not optimal, perhaps, but I've convinced myself that bribes are just another way of letting them choose.

Of course, youngsters aren't the only ones susceptible to manipulation. There are tons of books out there that teach us *How to Win Friends and Influence People*—that's the title of one of the bestselling self-help books of all time, written by Dale Carnegie in 1936. Another example is the popular *New York Times* essay "What Shamu Taught Me About a Happy Marriage," where writer Amy Sutherland shared how the techniques she learned from trainers of exotic animals helped her influence her own husband. She then wrote a book about using these techniques with all of the people in her life. Interestingly, she concluded that the only animal you can really transform is yourself.

Do Your Tao

I've found that the simplest way to change folks has nothing to do with them at all. Rather, it's about changing your own mindset—your perception of them.

In choosing to believe in others, we are often met with the best of what people have to offer, so I challenge you (and myself) to do this when you feel the crappiest. When the world feels bleak, when people seem mean, that is when you pull out your magic card of perception.

Choose to look for goodness and you will find it. Choose to see kindness, humanity, love. When you're fed up with your significant other, choose to see their vulnerability. When your kids seem like disobedient little devils, choose to see the lightness they can teach you. When someone is less than nice, see their underlying pain.

Because the opposite is also true—if you believe people are bastards, you will see more bastardly behavior than you could possibly stand. So, remember that we are all a bit of everything and decide to seek out light everywhere you go and in everyone you meet.

. . . .

choose to look for goodness and you will find it

. . . .

28

Zen-*ish*

Do you think you can take over the Universe and improve it?
I do not believe it can be done.

The world is a sacred vessel and it cannot be controlled.
You will only make it worse if you try—
it may slip through your fingers and disappear.

Allow your life to unfold naturally.
Know that it too is a vessel of perfection.

Just as you breathe in and breathe out,
there is a time for being ahead and a time for being behind;
a time for being in motion and a time for being at rest;
a time for being vigorous and a time for being exhausted;
a time for being safe and a time for being in danger.

To the Sage, all of life is a movement toward perfection.
He avoids extravagance, excess, and extremes.

—Tao Te Ching, Verse 29

That's why,

Let go of the oars, or, at least, loosen your grip on them (yours and
those of others, for that matter).
Allow your life to take you.

Pants, Dammit

We've all had the experience of undertakings that seem to go nowhere—relationships, jobs, projects that we refuse to let go of. It is
a human tendency to throw good money after bad because we fear
accepting all our wasted time and effort. So instead, we keep pushing
that expensive boulder up a hill, no matter how hard it is. Of course,
eventually the boulder rolls back down regardless. Sometimes we
end up squashed. Or emotionally, financially, physically bankrupt.

But what if we were to stop trying to push and control so much?
What if we shrugged and gave up when something felt off, and hung
on without all the fretting when it felt right? What if we remembered that nothing is ever wasted and that sometimes mistakes and
messes carry gifts, along with laughs? Not to mention that a straight
line would be so freaking boring!

"Can you wear size four jeans?" my friend recently asked me.

"Why?" I replied.

"They sent me the wrong size; maybe you'll like them."

"But, why don't you just send them back?" I wondered.

"Oh, girl, don't get me started," she said in her Texas drawl.
"This company's computers went batshit crazy and I spent thirty
minutes on the phone one night with some kid trying to get me new
pants. A woman in Atlanta got my pants and the pants I want to give
you were intended for a woman in Michigan."

She paused for breath.

"All of the women who got the wrong pants started talking to
each other via text (we had the phone numbers on the wrong mail-
ing slips *inside* the packages). When we got the right pants, we pho-
tographed them and sent the pictures to each other with the word
pants. They never did take back the wrong ones."

Feel free to replace "pants" with a romantic partner, or a job, a
house—you get the gist. Life can run circles around us sometimes.

But, perhaps, when the next curve ball hits you, you can just think "pants." Pants, dammit.

As it turned out, the wrong-sized pair my friend gave me fit like a glove from God.

The Garry Shandling Effect

Have you heard of Garry Shandling? He was quite the brilliant comedian whose '90s series *The Larry Sanders Show* seems ahead of its time. Adam and I rewatched it during that nebulous blob of a pandemic and the show held up like a fine wine—or whatever is funnier than a fine wine . . . aged cheese? But I really came to appreciate the man after watching a documentary by his protégé, Judd Apatow, called *The Zen Diaries of Garry Shandling*. In this film, we learn about Garry holistically: his heavy childhood in the shadow of his brother's death, the way he used his pain to fuel his comedy, and how it also got in his way. Most strikingly, we see how devoted he was to self-exploration and to evolving as a human being. Despite being a complicated, and at times, less than stable person, he worked very hard on bettering himself, and on coming to terms with life as it was—the good and the not so good. For example, *Transforming Problems into Happiness* by Lama Zopa Rinpoche was a book he swore by—a Buddhist read about the opportunities our difficulties present to us. His 2016 death was a big loss to his friends and to the world of comedy, but his diaries revealed that he wasn't scared of it in the slightest.

What I realized in watching this movie and in learning more about Shandling is that spirituality doesn't always look the way we think it should.

I used to kick myself for what I lacked spiritually, despite how much yoga I did and how many self-help books I read. I wanted to walk around with the air of an evolved being, spreading peace, wisdom, love, without a sound. I still dream of it: a priestess gliding with grace. It simply isn't who I am, though. And nothing is more frustrating than trying to be something you're not. On the other hand, embracing yourself will propel you forward.

I talk a lot (have I mentioned this already?). I overanalyze and fret and curse. Still, I am way more zen than I once was. I—like Garry Shandling, like you, like everyone—am always moving toward perfection, even when it doesn't seem like I am. There is no need to fight with my own overstimulated, zany nature. It is this frantic mind of mine that led me in search of peace in the first place. I suspect the same was true for Garry and for many a guru atop their spiritual throne.

If you, too, are less than zen, just shoot for zen-*ish*.

"There is a time for being ahead and a time for being behind; a time for being in motion and a time for being at rest." Our lives are always flowing, unfolding within a scheme we can't quite see. We simply need to let go of the oars from time to time.

Do Your Tao

Is there a person whose life you tend to meddle in—with the best intentions, of course—your child, your sibling, your friend? Well, this "Do Your Tao" tip is easy: Stop. Perhaps from your external vantage point it's easier to see where they're going wrong, how they can be happier or do better for themselves. Never mind. There's a time for being ahead and a time for being behind. Let them be behind—or less than happy, or confused, or whatever you think they are—for as long as they need to. Because you don't have the bigger picture; you don't know where their journey is taking them. Let them be exactly where they are without imposing your opinion.

Don't get me wrong, I understand how challenging this step-back approach is. My kids are still little and already I must force myself to abdicate control; of course, theirs are not yet big life decisions. But as a bossy older sister, keeping my mouth shut is a greater challenge. Alex, who is five years my junior, happens to be a sweetheart of a person. I used to feel the impulse to protect him, even if from himself, even when it wasn't my place. But once I realized that I didn't need to do this, that in fact it was his life to live, a huge weight was lifted off my shoulders. I still meddle sometimes; in my mind though, I've set him free.

Everyone has their own path and their own lessons to learn. Each one of us unfolds in our own perfect time.

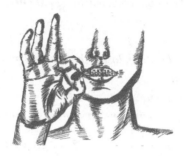

29

Peace Begins With You

When the world has the Way, horses roam freely.
When the world lacks the Way, warhorses are bred in the
  countryside.

There is no greater loss than losing the Way, no greater tragedy than
  discontentment;
contentment alone is enough.
The satisfaction of knowing one's true needs is eternal.

—TAO TE CHING, VERSE 46

Plus,

For the world to find the Way, you and I must find it within.

Changing the World

When you look at it from above, our world undeniably "lacks the Way." Many societies are puppeteered by warmongers and power-withholders. But a quick romp through our past reminds us that people have been less than at peace for, like, ever—with nature, with each other, with ourselves. The problem now is the closer we get to war, the greater the possibility of our extinction. In Lao Tzu's time, they bred warhorses; in our time it's drones and nuclear missiles. So when one government gets into a tiff with another, the stakes are higher than ever. Add on top of that the destruction of the Earth, unforeseen pandemics, and natural disasters . . . I mean how do we *not* go crazy with thoughts of our impending doom?

We are at a pivotal moment in history, when enlightenment must spread or else—and I happen to believe spiritual attunement, or the Way, will prevail. What we need to do is accept this power/responsibility: each one of us affects mass consciousness because we're all an integral part of it, and when enough of us intend peace, the world *will* change. Still, this work must begin from within.

Online there are many versions of a meme that asks, "Who wants change?" We all do! But when asked, "Who wants *to* change?" the answer becomes more complicated.

As President Trump's reign was coming to a close, an angry mob of his supporters who believed he should stay in power stormed the Capitol. In that same moment, there were families in my neighborhood detesting each other over the wearing or not-wearing of masks, even as their children tried to be friends. Just months prior, during nationwide Black Lives Matter demonstrations—and while my own town continued to diversify, becoming more and more the kind of place many of us wanted to raise our kids in—town old-timers dropped off unwelcoming T-shirts near the homes of newcomers, with writing which stunk of bigotry. Grown men and women were unable to reach for the love within (it is always there, even underneath anger and fear) and to communicate peacefully despite their differences. And I realized that what was going on in our country was just a macrocosm of the microcosm. So many people were clearly living in fear—fear of divergent opinions and beliefs, fear of *the other*, fear of not getting what they felt was owed to them.

The fact is, we cannot expect the world to change if we do not do so ourselves. For people to get along internationally, they need to find a way to get along within nations. For people to get along within a nation, they must do so within the towns and cities that comprise it. And for neighbors to live peacefully with one another, they must cultivate peace within themselves.

Changing Yourself

When it comes to social change, the fear we feel must be challenged and transformed, word by word, thought by thought. Because that is what all hatred is—fear. But when you learn to truly love yourself, your love naturally pours out for *the other*. More so, you realize the other *is* you—their joy is your joy, their pain, your pain. It is our job, then, to remind ourselves that racism is like spitting at God, as is anti-Semitism and homophobia. All forms of hatred are hatred of the Universe, a denial of the love of Source, the bottomless loss of the Way.

For, "there is no greater loss than losing The Way," the Tao tells us. And there's "no greater tragedy than discontentment."

It feels like the whole of modern society is built upon not-enoughness. Our capitalist culture is based on attainment and ambition; our spiritual one focuses on self-improvement. *How* do we cultivate contentment, then?

It helps me to remember that my primary relationship, my primary duty is to myself. There is no one I need to impress but me—and in fact, everyone else is already busy with their own goals and dreams. But, like many of us, I can get so busy striving, I forget to tell myself, "good job; I'm impressed," the way I would to my children or to my friends or spouse. I'm great at complimenting others, yet I treat myself like a robot sometimes, without so much as a pat on the back.

So, the question beckons: Can I love myself right now, with all of my incomplete missions and past fallacies? Can I be content with who I am and what I have?

I can, I decide. And so I become love.

It took me so long to be this happy-go-lucky person, though I've always played one on TV. What I mean is, I've always put on a smiley face, even prior to all the internal untangling. Now, though, it's a true representation of how I feel inside. Before the kids, before my best friend of a husband, I tapped into a place of eternity within myself; that is why I think I was able to meet him on the high-vibe plane he already inhabited, and to build a satisfying life together. Back then, I meditated and chanted, often in Sanskrit, without even understanding the words—but my intention was crystal clear: love, joy, freedom.

If this is all that happens to me for the rest of my life: I am a joyous person who raises her kids and laughs with her husband and loves her animals and nature and friends and strangers, I am content with that. *There is nothing lacking,* remember?

When we are able to discover and cultivate peace, we can carry it everywhere we go, spreading it like fairy dust. Each smile to a passerby, each warm word to a sullen friend is a speckle—I've seen it. And we've all seen people—both those who have nothing and those who have everything—shut down to the kindness of the world. We've seen them create drama and strife where there need not be any.

The more open we remain, the more we keep our egos in check, the more we are able to receive. The more intentional energy we spread, the more we are helping mass consciousness.

Do Your Tao

There is a simple mantra-mudra combination that I picked up from spiritual teacher Gabby Bernstein—she's posted it on her website and in YouTube videos, and I, in turn, have widely shared it too. It's accessible enough for my kids to remember. And a friend dealing with anxiety found it so helpful she made bracelets with its words. It can bring us back to a place of peace quickly, easily, and discreetly— ya know, for those who don't want to seem too *woowoo* in public. Ready?

The mantra (which is a phrase you repeat either silently or out loud) is "Peace begins with me." The mudra, or hand position, is touching your thumb to each of the other four fingers on your hand:

Thumb to index finger: *Peace*

Thumb to middle finger: *Begins*

Thumb to ring finger: *With*

Thumb to pinkie finger: *Me*

Technically, you're supposed to do it on both hands simultaneously, but why not be a badass like me and use just one? "Peace begins with me, peace begins with me," your fingers tap out. Because it does.

peace begins with me

30

Lay Down Your Arms

Weapons are the tools of violence and are detested by
all living things.

Weapons are the tools of fear.
Only as a last resort will a wise person use a deadly weapon.
Peace is his highest value; if the peace has been shattered, how can
he be content?
His enemies are not demons, but human beings like himself.
He doesn't wish them personal harm, nor does he glorify victory.
How could he delight in the slaughter of humanity?

He enters a battle gravely, with sorrow and with great compassion—
as if he were attending a funeral.

—TAO TE CHING, VERSE 31

And

How many needless lives have been lost to violence?
What can we do to decrease its imprint on humanity?
Let's remember: as within, so without.

Tools of Fear

What comes to your mind when you think *weapons*?

I think "weapons of mass destruction," which were used as an excuse to start a war, but which were never actually found. I think tanks and armies, which confound so many of us: on the one hand there are the soldiers who freed the victims of Nazi concentration camps and the ones that have delivered food to children in the crappiest situations; then there are those that caused and experienced so much suffering in Vietnam. And in my lifetime, the scarred soldiers who served in Iraq and in Afghanistan—*Why?* I keep thinking. *To what end?*

Yet before we even begin to face the issues of international relations and unnecessary wars, let us look closer to home—which brings us to guns.

Guns.

Gun.

I shudder at that three-letter word. And yet, the above verse from the Tao, written thousands of years ago, couldn't be more timely. Unfortunately, we haven't evolved beyond the regular use of weapons; only the weapons themselves have evolved: more bullets, more speed, faster evisceration of human life. Here we are in the 21st century with no concrete solution and not even a way to protect our children.

"We had a shelter-in-place drill in music today," Charlie said after coming home from kindergarten one afternoon. "We had to hide behind the piano, but not everyone could fit."

"Uhm," my face froze into a weird twitchy expression—it was unable to react quickly enough to what I was feeling and remembering. I mean, both my kids began regular safety drills in nursery school; they'd been practicing crouching in a corner since they were two—but those had been presented to them as games. It wasn't until I first entered an elementary school for Charlie's orientation that the reality of our nation's trauma hit me smack in the head. I wasn't alone; I saw the same panic on other parents' faces . . . and, the kids couldn't even fit behind the piano for God's sake.

In 2012, a sick young man shot and killed twenty-six people at Sandy Hook Elementary School in Newtown, Connecticut. He primarily used a legally purchased semi-automatic rifle. Twenty of the victims that day were children between six and seven years old.

Twenty bright-eyed, bushy-tailed little loves were eviscerated in minutes.

Upon first entering the quaint suburban elementary school in my neighborhood—a school much like Sandy Hook—my heart broke all over again for the lost youngsters, and for their parents, who, like me, loved their babies beyond all else and thought they were sending them to a safe environment for learning. Their grief is still palpable, as is our shame. Charlie is six years old as I write this and often when I look at her happy, innocent face, I catch myself imagining those departed six- and seven-year-olds of Sandy Hook— and let's not forget the six adults that died trying to protect them.

So, what do we do with all this sorrow? Do we just throw in the towel on humanity? It's awfully tempting sometimes.

Hundreds upon hundreds more shootings took place after Sandy Hook—in concerts and places of worship, and in other schools where we send our cherished youth. Our country has moved heaven and hell to fight terrorism, but has sadly done very little to decrease domestic gun violence, which is responsible for far more deaths. The power and influence of the National Rifle Association (and the money it donates to politicians) is indomitable. Still, we must keep working towards changing what seems unchangeable.

I pray that one day gun control laws will finally be enacted: gun buyback programs, thorough background checks, long waiting periods, to start. My motherly heart will forever mourn those lost children. I breathe and send light to their parents and grandparents, siblings and friends.

Sometimes change is slow, but I believe in its tide. I believe light will prevail.

Do Your Tao

I am not going to tell you what to do to help enact gun control. I figure you, too, have heard of organizations like Moms Demand Action. If you feel so inclined, read some of their findings, some of their stories. And next time there's an election, perhaps keep this issue in the forefront of your mind, as will I.

But just like we need to face violence here in America in order to understand it on a global scale, we also must address it in our homes and within ourselves.

Does violence exist within your own heart?

That's a rhetorical question; it is present in all of us (maybe with the exception of a handful of truly enlightened beings). Catch yourself the next time you're about to yell at your kids, your partner, someone at the store, or you're on the verge of honking and gesturing on the road—or when you're berating yourself. Take a pause, a breath, do the Peace thing from the last chapter. And when you notice it too late, like I sometimes do, apologize and start anew.

Whether it's directed inward or outward, violence *can* be alchemized. What is its root cause? Fear. And what is on the other side of fear? Love. Little by little, we can transform ourselves and the world. The process can feel slow as hell, but just the awareness itself is a step forward. In the end, we have no choice—we must lay down our arms.

31

Break Free

The Tao is nameless, simple, subtle.
If powerful men and women could remain centered in it, the world
would become a paradise;
people would have no need for laws because the laws would be
written in their hearts.

The world is nothing but the glory of the Tao expressed through
different names and forms.
One who sees the things of this world as being real and self-existent
has lost sight of the truth;
to him, every word becomes a trap, every thing becomes a prison.

One who knows the truth that underlies all things lives in this world
without danger;
to him, every word reflects the Universe, every moment brings
enlightenment.

All things end in the Tao,
just as all streams and rivers flow into the sea.

—TAO TE CHING, VERSE 32

The takeaway:

So many of us live in a prison of our own making (and judge those
who don't).
We create entire systems that imprison us in one way or another.
Let's stop—one single person, one leader, one organization at a
time.

Imprisonment/Freedom

Though liberty is something I mostly take for granted these days, I'd like to think I have an inherent understanding of a freedomless existence. Hailing from the USSR, my family wasn't allowed to practice their religion or to travel to places that interested them. My young parents couldn't read books the government deemed dangerous or listen to the music they longed for (like the hairy, dangerous Beatles, as Soviet leaders called them).

"We used to play less than partisan songs," my dad told me about a band he had in college, "and we were a hit."

"Really?" I asked.

"Yes, but we were warned the KGB was after us; they'd throw us in jail," he said.

"So what did you do?"

"We stopped playing," he shrugged.

He and my mom left everything they knew, two kids and a *babushka* in tow, to follow their dream of living freely. We were refugees, then immigrants, then citizens. And, yet, I still need reminders to appreciate my freedom and to revel in it.

I guess it's easy for us to get caught up with family life, our circle of friends and frenemies, politics, the news, you name it . . . we tend to live myopic lives. So it's a small miracle that I escaped my own little bubble and got a very healthy dose of perspective from behind bars.

Freedom/Imprisonment

Several years ago, in a very New York writing group where folks divulged the wildest of experiences, I met an incredible person who runs a program for incarcerated juveniles and women. She once spent time in jail herself and gives back with classes in which she teaches forgotten souls to tell their stories.

One evening, I tagged along with her to the women's prison at Rikers Island—by way of an hours-long bureaucratic labyrinth—bringing with me a deck of Tao Te Ching cards and my white liberal yearning to help.

"Be like water," I recited, reading them my take on one of my favorite verses from the Tao, "Flow over shit and say, 'Fuck this, I'm water.'"

They chuckled.

I told them they could drip slowly or vaporize and reemerge as fog if they so chose. I wanted them to remember they are fluid, ever-transforming, that the bars which enclose them are but a physical constraint.

They wanted me to know that it's the little things they miss most.

They spoke of their heavy pasts—heavier than most of us can imagine—so dense in fact that they're not for me to divulge; I hope one day they will share these stories with anyone who will listen. And they lit up when reciting the simplest pleasures we take for granted but which they dream of nightly: grass, trees, the open sky, french fries, their children.

One woman had two girls like I do, just slightly older. She had lived a life filled with trauma and in a way found jail to be a reprieve. There, she rediscovered her strong self; she found the willpower to fight for her freedom.

I had not expected the appreciation for life to be quite so vivid within those prison walls. The women I met had endured so much, and yet, I witnessed their hope and their longing for life's joy—which so often gets dulled for us, the "free" ones, by the unimportant details of the rat race.

What's important and what isn't? I now ask myself, though probably not often enough. I long to see the truth, and to not get stuck in imprisoning thoughts and beliefs. I refuse to let the minutia of the world close me in (I mean most of the time; a few days a month, my hormones choose differently). I feel I owe it to those who are less free to revel in my liberties, in nature, in my children. We all do. And we owe them a chance to start anew, without judgment for their past—not to mention an improved criminal justice system. Freedom, after all, is reciprocal: when you free another from your decrees and expectations, you free yourself.

Do Your Tao

Take some time to fully experience the liberties missed by the women behind bars: fresh air, blue or gray or cloudy skies, snow or sunshine on your face—it's all wonderful, really. Find time amidst your daily hustle to take it in. Enjoy your meal, laugh with your children, your dog, your friends. Express your thoughts. Be unabashedly yourself. Take pleasure in being alive, with the agency to choose your goals and destinations.

If you are going through a dark time, you can be sure the sun will reemerge tomorrow or the day after. Still, allow for the beauty of tonight's moon.

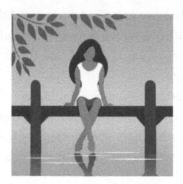

32

Earthing

*Living in oneness, the sky is clear, the Earth is at peace, and all
    creatures live joyfully upon it.
When man interferes with the Tao, the sky becomes filthy, the Earth
    depleted,
equilibrium crumbles, creatures become extinct.*

*The Master views the parts with compassion because he understands
    the whole.
He doesn't shine like a precious gem, but lets himself be shaped by
    the Tao—
as rugged, as common as a stone.
He chooses to practice humility by living in accordance with the
    whole universe.*

—TAO TE CHING, VERSE 39

May I add?

The Master knows she is as good as anyone and better than
no one.

Baby Steps

So, I am no expert on climate change, pollution, or the Earth's eco-systems. I don't think I'm much of an expert on anything to be honest, except for spiritual awakening. But the fact that Lao Tzu's words have proven unquestionable thousands of years later is obvious to me. Man has in fact interfered with the natural order of things. He has depleted the Earth and driven creatures to extinction. Because for much of modernity, we have not been aligned with the goodness of our planet; nor have we remained humble with the power we've been given.

And yet, I watch young kids pick up litter left behind in the park. My girls listen intently as Adam or I explain why we don't step on bugs or ants, why we don't squash spiders but rather carry them out. Hope is not lost. Our children will do better than we have. And we can all commit to improvement, little by little—in moments of simply doing the right thing.

Barbara Marx Hubbard, activist and author of *Conscious Evolution: Awakening the Power of Our Social Potential,* explains it perfectly. She likens us—the ones who are waking up to our power, potential, and responsibility—to the imaginal cells within a caterpillar that eventually transform its disintegrating body into a butterfly. So even if the things we *can* do for our planet seem minuscule, Hubbard's analogy reminds us that when enough of us imprint a new way of living, the world will, in fact, transform.

"What does it matter if one person recycles or not?" I used to think, until I understood that each little correction to our unbalanced system is worthy. These small acts add up: recycling, eating less meat, adopting animals from a shelter rather than purchasing them, treating those animals like the majestic creatures they are, as well as all the other animals we encounter in our lives—the squirrels, the pigeons, the mice, the bugs. Seriously, even cockroaches. I get you end up squashing them sometimes; but, like, offer an apology while you do so.

There are thousands of little actions we can take to better coexist with our earth.

Living in harmony with oneself is a good start, and then spreading that sense of peace and balance to every relationship, every interaction, every action. If each of us does our best, we can bring ourselves back into alignment. Change happens one person, one pure choice at a time.

Humility

I don't particularly like to stand out or "shine like a gem," and yet a part of me craves to be acknowledged. *How could both truths exist in one person?* I wonder.

"The Master views the parts with compassion because he understands the whole."

As a child, I felt lesser than, like I didn't belong in this superior American world. But as I grew, along with my breasts, I became more and more aware of my assets. Throughout college, in a fog of depression, I thought I was better than everybody—smarter, more sophisticated, prettier—too good. Too delicate, too vulnerable, too special. So righteous, in fact, that my own best friend couldn't stand me (we took a nearly two-year-long hiatus). I glittered like a cold, lonely jewel, dressed to the nines in form-fitting, low-cut, high-heeled ensembles; it was a surface perfection which only masked my pain.

Now, as a tired mom, often inches away from haggard, when I look at people with seemingly perfect lives or exteriors, I wonder how much lies behind the curtain. We all have our days—or years—when we are barely keeping it together, but only some of us show it. I'm finally (mostly) comfortable being exactly who I am, and when I'm not comfortable, I choose to be real anyway.

It took a couple decades, a few twists and turns for me to realize I am but a stone, just like everyone is. Because our truest uniqueness comes from embracing our ordinary humanity, our crooked stories, our faults and sore spots, as they chisel away at us.

The Tao Te Ching suggests that humility is a practice—a constant reminder to oneself: "I am no better than anyone," "I am as good as anyone."

I first heard this sentiment from my teenage boyfriend's mother. She emigrated to New York from Italy when she was eleven years old and never went to school again. She worked as a cook at a community center, took care of her children and a gaggle of nieces and nephews, and smoked her cigarettes. I don't know if there were parts of herself she hadn't explored but wished to—I always felt a sense of sadness beneath her life of service and warmth. She was tired, like many women of her generation were and still are. But her goodness always shined through.

"As good as anyone; better than no one"—that, to me, is the essence of humility.

Do Your Tao

What is one small, humble thing you can do for your planet right now?

Perhaps, it's purchasing a reusable bottle to fill with water daily in order to cut down on plastic, or picking up litter when you see it left behind. You can commit to eating less meat—some scientists say decreasing meat consumption would be the single biggest way to help the planet. This doesn't mean becoming a vegetarian, but simply eating less of it (beef and pork, especially). "Less" can mean no more than once a day, for instance, or weekends only; improving our balance with the Earth need not be an all-or-nothing endeavor. If each of us makes even small changes, the effects will be large indeed.

33

"Dear God, Dear Hashem, Dear Lord"

Return is the movement of the Tao.
Yielding is the application of the Tao.

All things arise from worldly interactions, or being.
Being arises from emptiness or non-being.

—Tao Te Ching, Verse 40

And

We are always in the process of returning, whether we yield
to life or not . . .
but yielding feels so much better.

Praying

I think of the "return" Lao Tzu speaks of here as our constant movement forward in the circle of life, which, being a circle, eventually brings us back to the non-being from which we began. "Yielding" is the way to go with the direction of this return—by allowing, by giving in to life itself, rather than bucking against it. The former is a given; the latter, an invitation.

When I was a kid living in Brooklyn, I badly wanted magic. I'd lost control of my circumstances, finding myself in a new country where I no longer had a clear place. My confidence wavered. Without planning to, by middle school I began to pray. Every night before going to bed, I would stand in front of my window mulling over my circumstances, as I'd recite my self-made incantation: "Baruch Ata Adanoi, Dear God, Dear Hashem, Dear Lord," followed by my wishes. In mixing together the beginning of Hebrew prayers I'd occasionally hear with whatever other names of God I could think of, I thought I was covering all the bases.

I've since realized that all of life is a prayer, every thought, every word, every action—and frankly, some of what we inadvertently pray for is crap. Yet, middle school—a period which is so confusing for many of us (and also high school, and perhaps college . . . and, in my case, my twenties)—that precarious moment between childhood and adulthood is when I think the lot of us is praying extra hard, even if we don't realize it. We pray for safety or for excitement, to blossom or to hang onto innocence, and we yearn, beg, plead for acceptance and for love.

"Baruch Ata Adanoi, Dear God, Dear Hashem, Dear Lord, please let him notice me," I'd whisper in the dark.

I began sneaking makeup out of my mom's pocketbook and asked her to teach me how to shave my legs and bleach my 'stache.

"Baruch Ata Adanoi, Dear God, Dear Hashem, Dear Lord, please let me not get made fun of anymore."

I talked back to some of my tormentors, finally standing up for myself. I began using curse words. And badass lip-liner.

"Baruch Ata Adanoi, Dear God, Dear Hashem, Dear Lord," I'd chant, often not even knowing what to ask for—just gazing at the couple stars I could make out from the depths of my crowded borough. I wanted to feel a connection to something greater. I searched for it constantly.

all of life is a prayer

One day after school, I watched Deepak Chopra talk about spirituality on *The Oprah Winfrey Show*. I don't remember the details of their conversation, only that by the time my dad came home from work that night, I was sitting cross-legged, staring straight ahead. My eyes were focused on a button that was tied to a string which I'd suspended from a wall light, as I willed it to move.

Eventually, we left that apartment for a house in the burbs, and then that house for another house. And then I squatted in one room or another for years, until I found my home in Adam and then with Adam.

Still, a part of me will always remain in a Brooklyn apartment, a determined little girl who knows she can move a button with her mind.

Yielding

Unlike human determination, the yielding part, which is based in trust, doesn't come naturally to most of us. It is the release of the reins, the allowing of people and circumstances to be as they are. It's barely an afterthought in our world, where we are taught to plow on and to *make* things happen, and yet, it's the most pleasant way of being.

This ability to yield does reside deep within us, even if we have forgotten it. It's sort of like when we take a deep inhale, we suddenly remember how good it feels to breathe—that is also how it feels to yield.

And so I remind myself to yield to my career as it unfolds outside of my plans, in ways I couldn't possibly foresee, and to my marriage, which shifts and flows freely if Adam and I let it (even allowing it to dip when it does). I aim—sometimes I struggle—to yield to my daughters who are the strongest of beings, uncontrollable the more I try to control them.

I want to yield to the Tao, rather than to my own ego. I want us all to yield to miracles.

Do Your Tao

Think of a situation in your life that could benefit from you yielding: A battle of wills at work or at home? An unwanted circumstance? Opposing views? The next time you find yourself there, stop fighting, choose again. Take that deep inhale to remind yourself how to give way, how to allow the situation to be what it is. Then withdraw, preserve your energy, and see what happens. In the least, your inhale will be followed by an exhale. Make *that* your prayer—the choice to breathe rather than to fight—a living prayer.

34

Not of This World

She who follows the way of the Tao will draw the world to her steps.
She perceives the universal harmony, even amid great pain,
because she has found peace in her heart.

Music and sweets are passing pleasures,
but how bland and insipid are the things of this world when one
    compares them with Tao!
One tastes, but the sweetness turns bitter.
One sees, but the colors grow faint.
One hears, but the sound fades into silence.

One may look for fulfillment in this world but her longings will never
    be exhausted;
the only thing she ever finds is that she herself is exhausted.

—TAO TE CHING, VERSE 35

Or

Remember that worldly pleasures can't fulfill you (not consistently,
at least).
The more sensitive you are, the more you need to connect to the
Great Power within.
And when everything seems dark, please keep going;
it's not the end—just a tunnel towards the light.

Lost

What happens to those of us who are overly sensitive but are unable to find the release, the freedom, the evolution of escaping our problems? This is a question that haunts me, it lives within me and also in this book.

"There but by the grace of God, go I," I think. Because not everyone is fortunate enough to find their way.

"I'm so sorry, auntie," I mumbled to my childhood friend's mother, "I'm sorry, uncle," as I wondered if in some alternate universe it could've been me inside that wooden box. I hadn't seen them in years—his parents—our families had a falling out for reasons I can't quite piece together. They all seem so ridiculous now; we, humans, can be ridiculous. He never walked the familial party lines anyway, but now he is gone, and with him any connection to his brood that I thought was also my brood once. But, that was lifetimes ago.

This lost boy and I—the one who died by suicide a couple years ago—immigrated to America together, both of us children leaving everything we knew and waiting in purgatory to be granted asylum in the land of plenty. Our families awaited our fates in Europe side by side and then simultaneously settled down in New York.

For me, the displacement was shocking. Still, as I held back tears in my overcrowded inner-city classroom, I vowed to keep my sadness to myself. My parents—and his parents—were working so hard to put down roots in this country, to build a life, a future. I feel like we, the children, carried the grief of our lost selves in silence. I had a secret world of blue within me for many years. As my mental health wavered, so did his.

For lack of a better word, I was a loser, or so I saw myself—a screwup. I lived with my mom and dad well into adulthood (like many non-Americans, now that I think about it). I couldn't figure out relationships. I scared countless guys away, then tried to stalk them into submission. Even friendships slipped through my hands, different versions of un-friending and being un-friended.

I wonder if he also saw himself this way.

I know that as I worked towards a state of zen—I'm still working—he searched as well. He practiced martial arts and played the bass. I found me a good American man and became a mom in a good American town, and almost forgot the refugee pain that riddled me for half a lifetime.

But then, the lost boy threw in the towel and a sea of Soviet immigrants descended upon his Brooklyn grave. Amidst the rays of the autumn sun, we wept and exchanged wordless embraces, trying to offer something, anything to his shattered parents, his young wife folded like a paper doll.

"Amen," we whispered when the rabbi said his prayers. What else was there to say?

This boy, with countless friends, felt all alone in the end. He hadn't figured out how to heal, but I don't know why he decided to stop trying; no one will ever know. He'd flailed between careers, between identities even, like I had. We became strangers more or less, but in a way, wasn't he a stranger to everyone?

He had a child, a girl. We got together with our daughters once; he was the most doting of fathers.

Found

And so we each stood at the cemetery with our memories of him, a silent *Why?* permeating the air. His sister wrote him a letter filled with regret and love that transcends death, I hope. In the end, as he returned to the Tao, he gave us all a gift—a spark of its light amidst the darkness. And every one of us, displaced children and tired adults living in a country that's not quite theirs, can do with it as they wish.

I took this light home to my girls. It kept me up at night after I put them to bed. I wrapped it around myself like a heavy, woolen scarf. I called the friends I'd been meaning to call for ages.

If I am being honest with myself, I'm not a hundred percent certain I was made for this world either. I've never been able to master the adult things: career, order, good silverware. But that's okay.

"She who follows the way of the Tao will draw the world to her steps."

Perhaps, we don't need to focus so intensely on this outward realm after all. Instead, we can cultivate inner peace and allow our own little world to assemble around it. I wish for everyone like me (all of us drifters) to find a way to create a nook where we can flourish, to keep trying—even when it feels like we aren't made for this world. *Especially* then.

Do Your Tao

Those of us who've made it back from the dark side have the advantage of now truly appreciating the light. Let's recommit to keeping it lit within ourselves and others. Today, call someone you haven't in a while. Or do something kind for a neighbor who seems lonely—all it takes is a friendly chat to make another's day.

Let's also remember those who haven't returned from the abyss and never will—we send them eternal love.

But, you, my dear reader, you are here; you have all you need within you; keep swimming towards the light.

35

The Wordless Chapter

The gentlest thing in the world overrides the hardest.
That which has no substance enters where there is no space.
Thus we can appreciate the value of not pushing or contriving.

Wordless teaching and not contriving—
certainly there is nothing greater under Heaven.

—Tao Te Ching, Verse 43

Because,

The gentleness of inviting peace will overcome the hardness of life . . . and how words make you feel is more important than the words themselves.

Why Words?

Clearly, I teach *with* words. And I listen to and learn from others who teach with words. And yet, there is a wordless state we must all experience in order to evolve spiritually. So why are all these words even necessary?

Well, the truth is they are not. (I probably should've told you that before you picked up this book.) Babies, for example, before they have the ability to speak or understand language, exist in a state of grace. They don't contrive. They simply are. But they do not remain thus because that is not the plan. That's not why we came here to this physical plane. Otherwise, we could have just remained in the non-physical, right?

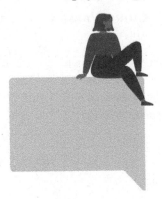

We came here for a reason, which each of us must discover, create, or experience in our own unique way. And en route we forget our original oneness.

We accrue ideas and fears, beliefs and neuroses—some necessary, much of them extraneous. And so I guess the words and the teachings exist and keep being spoken and written in order to remind ourselves of who we are, who we have always been. By *feeling* that knowledge, that power while here in our physical form . . . well . . . who knows what we could achieve? Anything. Everything. I'll tell you in my next book. Or, better yet, I'll beam it to you or you to me.

Running Away

Unlike babies, I do not exist in a state of grace. And so I run away from home sometimes. Depending on the season and the presence, or not, of a pandemic, I choose where to go. I may run away to a Kundalini yoga class or to my little Italian coffee shop, for a bike ride in the woods or a walk around the block. When I find myself at my wits' end, I know I must run—not because my daughters and husband are so challenging (which they can be) and not because I get bored (which happens too, though rarely), not even because I am tired, which I usually am if I stop to think about it. I run because I need to get away from myself.

You know when you're stuck in a negative mental loop? I am never going to achieve anything, the odds are stacked against me, I don't even know what I'm doing, who the hell do I think I am? And on and on and on. This timeworn self-doubt and despair shock me with their reappearance—a sleeping giant seemingly awakened by stress and exhaustion, though it's always lurking, waiting for a chance to weigh in. Or it can be as simple as undefined anxiety roaring inside my chest that commands me to seek out Spirit, to run for the mystical hills.

I've learned that if it is remotely possible, one must heed one's need to escape. When your soul screams "Go," whether you're stuck in the office or behind the stove, find the opportunity ASAP—even if it's only for ten minutes or ten breaths—do it. You may not believe that any worthy shift is possible in such a short time, but it is. From feeling flat like stepped-on poop to feeling like a goddess, thanks to just a bit of breath, Tao, nothingness. The gentleness of inviting peace will always overcome the hardness of life.

We are not our thoughts, we are not our egos, we are not our negativity. We aren't even our dreams and aspirations.

We are part of eternal God energy—that which has no physical substance—and gods have no need to push, to fight, or to struggle. Gods *are*, they *be*, they shine softly, speak softly (not me, I'm the *loud* exception that proves the rule). They exist and move about naturally—like air, like water, like breath itself.

Choosing Light

As Martin Luther King Jr. said in his 1957 *Loving Your Enemies* sermon, "Darkness cannot drive out darkness; only light can do that. Hate cannot drive out hate; only love can do that."

We must remember his words today, in our speedy, anxious, tumultuous modern society—ever trigger-ready and tit-for-tat. The gentlest thing overcomes the hardest. But first, we need to cultivate this understanding within ourselves, and in our homes and relationships—every shift affects the unified field or mass consciousness, so let us not underestimate our effect on the world.

If we encounter someone rude in our day-to-day lives, it is so tempting to snap back with spite. Yet, gentleness or non-action is also a choice.

To reprimand our children when they misbehave—to raise our voices or enforce punishments—that is one choice. (Whenever I do that, Charlie cries, "You don't love me anymore," making me eat my words.) Is there a way to interact with our kids more softly, to remember their still-developing brains and personalities, even when they drive us mad?

And when we berate ourselves for wasted time, laziness, disorganization—and for our inability to calmly handle our children—can we just stop? Sure we are flawed with plenty of room for improvement; sure we strive to be better. Still, in order to be more gentle in the world, we must start by being gentle to ourselves—a self-pat on the back rather than constant criticism, and *When I align with the energy of the Universe, I can do anything*, rather than *Who do I think I am?*

Do Your Tao

The next time you find yourself in a negative loop—or if you're there right now—*stop*. Drop everything as soon as you can. Your primary goal at that moment is to disrupt the negative thought pattern. Go for a walk if you can and breathe deeply, and if that's not an option, hide in the closet or in the bathroom for a moment and take in stillness. Inhale, pause, exhale, expanding your belly on the in breath and letting it contract on the out. Remember that you are not your thoughts—you can observe them but you don't have to believe them.

I offer you this Kundalini blessing which is used to close out each class—hear it as you breathe:

May the long time sun
Shine upon you,
All love surround you,
And the pure light within you
Guide your way on.

Before I had any idea where this little song or blessing came from, it brought me comfort. As I was put on bed rest during my first pregnancy, I reached out to an acquaintance—a yoga teacher— who had been on bed rest for much of her own pregnancy. That is the song she sent me, which I'd listen to over and over while lying alone in the hospital, baby in belly. I'd close my eyes and know that she and I would be okay, as I know you will be.

· ·

breathe

· ·

36

Be Responsible for Your Energy

The Tao gives birth to one.
One gives birth to two (yin and yang).
Two gives birth to three (as in heaven, earth, man, or mind, body,
    soul).
The Three gives birth to all things as we know them.
This interplay of forces fills the Universe,
yet only at the still-point between the breathing in and the
    breathing out,
can one be in perfect harmony.

Who knows what fate may bring:
one day your loss may be your fortune, one day your fortune may be
    your loss.
The age-old maxim that others teach, I also teach:
"As you plant, so you reap."
Know this to be the foundation of my teachings.

—Tao Te Ching, Verse 42

In practice,

Fate is a mixed bag, but we can flow with it and aim to be present.
In the now, we become aware of our kind or shitty undercurrents;
then we can be intentional with our energy.

Future—What Future?

We don't ever really know what's in store for us down the line—our modern-day pandemic proved as much. Never in a million years would most of us have predicted it (well Bill Gates might have; but most of us, not so much). Yet there we were, suddenly standing in line just to enter a grocery store—a sight I thought I'd never see in America. In that moment, I viscerally recalled the long Soviet lines for goods I had once lived with, and how my mom begged for a chance to purchase hot dogs and was denied, and how little selection there was in my early years. These memories somehow helped me. *I had lived this way for the first decade of my life, I can do it again,* I figured. My loss—or lack, in this case: I had close to nothing material to start with—became my fortune.

It was as if my body remembered and reset itself accordingly. It's not that I handled this crisis perfectly by any means; it's just that losing the familiar didn't shake my core—been there, done that, I guess.

The Still Point of the Turning World

Since we cannot foretell or control external circumstances, how do we not panic? How do we accept uncertainty?

By tapping into the depths of Now, the Tao suggests, by falling into that gap between breathing in and breathing out. As philosopher Eckhart Tolle wrote in his book *The Power of Now,* suffering comes from resisting the present moment, and so that's where salvation must lie as well.

Think about it: in this very instance as you're reading these very words, your life is exactly as it is. And as imperfect or undesirable as some of your circumstances may be, right this second, you might surprisingly be feeling okay. In fact, as you focus on your breath, your problems cease; you simply are. You have entered the opening of presence. Only from here is enlightenment, healing, and transcendence possible.

When you stop overthinking, over-feeling, and over-wanting, you kind of forget about your human self—the personality with all its needs and hurts, the one we are all so sick of sometimes—and instead you align with a Higher Self, which spans way beyond your human form. You go from being a physical body to being nobody, from being somewhere to being nowhere . . . or everywhere, depending on how you look at it. This temporary retreat from the physical world returns you to your origin—to the Tao, the black hole, oneness.

This is a state I aim to embody at least once in a while—a practice in which I close my eyes (or keep them open) and simply exist, even if but briefly. It can be as effortless as reminding myself to *be here now*.

"Oh, look at that scrumptious cheek talking a mile a minute," I say to myself while listening to my daughter.

"There's the Hudson River flowing into the horizon," I try to notice.

"Breathe in, pause, breathe out," I tell myself—because that moment of harmony is always available to us.

Beyond Thoughts

You reap what you sow, the last part of this verse is telling us. "Know this to be the foundation of my teachings." Karma, in other words, or the Law of Attraction. You get back from the Universe that which you put in, energetically speaking. And more esoterically, since You, God, the Universe is all there is, you either poison yourself or bless yourself with the vibes you put forth—or for many of us, it's something in between.

Dr. Jill Bolte Taylor, a neuroanatomist who had a stroke in the left side of her brain, realized that when she couldn't speak or communicate with others, she was extremely sensitive to their energy field, feeling it immediately. This information—coming from a scientist, no less—helped me realize that I'm responsible for the energy I bring to each moment, each situation, each relationship. Sometimes I create magic with this knowledge; other times, I create mayhem in spite of it.

The thing is, underneath our words and actions is vibration, an unnameable field that others perceive and respond to. Understanding this can be exciting, empowering, and also alarming. Because when you don't like someone or you judge them or are mad at them, they feel it on some level, even if you're nothing but lovely to their face. And people can feel it when you have a wall up, regardless of how friendly you are with your words. Basically, everything within you corresponds to or manifests as something outside of you. Most of the time, it's a muddled mix of good and bad.

Living intentionally means being responsible not just for what you say and do, but even for the subtle vibes you put out. And there's no pressure—you are allowed to have that wall up whenever and with whomever you want—just know that what you feel towards another is felt by them as well. And that harmony is available to you no matter what's going on.

"To experience peace does not mean that your life is always blissful. It means that you are capable of tapping into a blissful state of mind amidst the normal chaos of a hectic life," wrote Dr. Taylor in her book *My Stroke of Insight*.

Do Your Tao

Find time today to reach for the blissful state Dr. Taylor and so many teachers speak of. It's not always easy to do, of course. When you feel like shit, being told to get blissful is like a cruel joke. But it's the upward trajectory that's important—the ability to take charge of your energy and emotions. On days when you feel off (or worse), just aim for a slightly better energy field—even if you go from waves of ennui to a smidgen of hope, you're moving towards possibility. In fact, Abraham—the collective spiritual wisdom channeled by Esther Hicks—lays out an entire emotional scale to help us track our movement. If you go from depression to anger, you're moving in the right direction—from anger towards disappointment, from disappointment to boredom, from boredom to hopefulness, and so on, until you end up in the immersive joy, love, and freedom of the Universe.

You can't feel peachy all the time, but you *can* observe yourself.

Treat yourself like the grandest machine on earth—when you need some tuning or downtime, take it. If you have a serotonin deficiency like me, or another brain idiosyncracy, be mindful. Watch yourself. Talk yourself out of ruts, not into them. And be aware of the energy you're bringing to your life and to the world. Remember that you have the power to shift it.

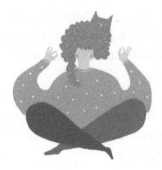

37

On Death and Dying

Anyone who is born dies.
If thirteen people are born, all thirteen will eventually die.
From birth to life, from life to death,
The Great Earth will afford them places to live and to die.
Why is this so?
Because the mind clings to this passing world.

But I hear there are those so sure of life that wild animals keep clear.
Weapons turn from them on the battlefield, rhinoceroses have no
   place to horn them, tigers find no place for claws, and soldiers
   have no place to thrust their blades.
Why is this so?
Because they dwell where death cannot enter.

Realize your essence.

                      —TAO TE CHING, VERSE 50

Or

You're born, you live, you die.
But the greater You is neither born, nor can it die,
it simply is—always.
So what is there to fear?

Death.

"Mommy, don't die, mommy, don't die," Gigi, then three, serenaded me one beautiful spring day.

I did a double-take. "What did you say?"

"Yikes," my husband added.

"It's my song," she told us, continuing to hum it in her sweet voice. "Do you like it?"

My grandmother had died two weeks prior; my other *babushka* was gravely ill. Neighbors' loved ones had also passed away, and everybody in sight wore masks to ward off contagion. Still, *Why is she singing this?* I thought.

For parents of young children like ours, it was hard to accept that they viscerally felt what was going on in the world (they always do) despite our efforts to shield them.

"Hiking is even more fun than the playground," we'd tell them when playgrounds were off limits. And "Frozen yogurt won't be closed forever . . ." "Isn't it nice you get to be home with your family for now?" Little beige lies mixed in with what we hoped was the truth.

So I was shocked the first time I heard my youngster tell her stuffed animals that they can't go anywhere because of COVID.

"How do you know that word?" I asked.

"Because I know," she told me, "because I'm smart."

And because she's smart, she easily understood that whenever our cat Regis brought a mouse or a chipmunk to our doorstep, that creature was no longer with us, so to speak. "It died and then it was dead," she'd say. However, she also believed these animals could be brought back to the land of the living. When a dead deer was spotted in the woods, she was certain "someone will turn him back to life."

According to parenting experts, we should correct kids' misconceptions about death. Except how can we possibly know what's a *mis*conception?

I didn't think she was that wrong about the deer—theoretically, his body did fertilize the soil and facilitated the growth of trees or moss or mushrooms. Plus, maybe the deer returned as a bear. How could I know what was in store for his afterlife? At best, I agreed with her; at worst, I was utterly confused.

The first years of my own life were shaped by the militantly atheist Soviet Union. After we immigrated here, Hebrew school mystified me. I knew we'd survived the Holocaust, but when I first asked my parents if they believed in God, they answered, "*Nyet*" in unison. Eventually, I leaned towards Eastern philosophy; maybe I always had. I remember inadvertently making my young friend cry when I told her about reincarnation.

"So my mother won't be my mother?" she asked.

I paused, then said "No" matter-of-factly. I didn't want to admit that her question had caught me off guard. She then rushed to call said mother in tears to come pick her up.

If I could go back in time, I would answer, "I'm not sure," and maybe add, "I think your mama will always be with you in some form," because I've grown to value mystery over black-and-white declarations, and humility over self-assuredness. I still believe reincarnation is likely. And it seems I'm in good company: children.

After my friend lost her mother to COVID, her son sweetly announced that she would come back as a baby . . . I hope she has.

And even though it freaked me out at first, I've accepted Gigi's fascination with death.

"Baba Klara is not going to get a shot?" she asked about the vaccine, referring to my deceased grandma.

"No," I said.

"Because she is dead?"

"Yes."

This line of thinking is expressed regularly in our house. When the girls are playing Barbies, I overhear "Let's pretend the mom is dead," for example, or they ask me, "You will die before us, right?"

"Yes," I answer, adding a mental *God, I hope so.*

I get it. Death actually is fascinating if we don't sweep it under the rug—especially when we look at it not as the end of being, but as a transition.

Death?

Our relationship with death here in the West seems less than comfortable, which makes sense—loss hurts; the unknown is scary. I do think, however, that we can strive to improve it, being that the physical experience of death is inevitable for every living thing. It is a part of nature, and since humans are also a part of nature, we are actually one: life—that is, us in human form, and death—that is, the end of this form.

We are life, but we are also death.

Yet the Tao tells us of those so certain of life that they dwell "where death cannot enter." They see themselves as much more than mere human bodies, so rather than dying the way we understand it, they simply shed these bodies.

 My girls tell me frequently that before they came here to be my daughters, they were waiting in the sky. I suspect there is truth to their story, though who knows what "the sky" actually is. We are born, we live, we die, but the greater We is never born at all. It is. Always. In one form or another—in forms we probably can't yet comprehend. How can we not find that fascinating?

Do Your Tao

What are your earliest memories of death? Do you remember when you first heard about this concept. Because in a way, death is a learned concept. Usually, it creeps into our psyche at a youngish age, before we are able to feel things out for ourselves—others' views of death become our own; how we think about it is shaped by the reactions of the adults around us. If there is a tragic or sudden loss involved—trauma, grief—we learn to fear death or to hate it or to push away the very idea of it. We may become interested in death, like my kid had, but this too is pushed away and discouraged—I know I am guilty of changing the topic as quickly as possible. How can I discuss it with my child if I haven't discussed it with myself?

So let us aim to take control of our relationship with death. First we need to acknowledge our fears, then we can negotiate them within. You can write it, think it, speak it—you can do it over and over again or find freedom in an instant. The point is, when you re-frame death, you free yourself to live.

Here I go:

I am so scared of death because I dread the idea of being sep-arated from my children. And, when I think about it in relation to anybody else, it feels like a bad omen. But then I tell myself that I *cannot* be separate from my girls, nor can my thoughts make another live or die. In fact, my relationship with anyone I'm close to will con-tinue after their or my physical passing.

This is a back-and-forth process for me of realizing my essence, as the Tao calls it. When I am able to move past the fear, death becomes a benevolent unknown.

Try your own reconfiguration of the death concept. And for a mind blowing afternoon, read up on NDEs (near-death experi-ences), check out the Netflix documentary, *Surviving Death*, or Anita Moorjani's book *Dying to Be Me*. There are so many out-of-the-box stories to shake up what we think we know. Why not let them?

CREATION

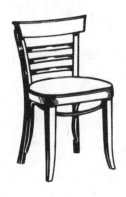

38

Success Sucks (Sometimes)

Success is as dangerous as failure,
and we are often our own worst enemy.

Whether you go up the ladder or down it, your position is shaky.
When you stand with your two feet on the ground, you will always
keep your balance.

See the world as yourself; have faith in the way things are.
Then you can truly care for all things.

—TAO TE CHING, VERSE 13

Or

Not even your greatest dream come true will rid you of your
demons;
that's why God invented therapy and self-help books!

Hollywood Fantasy

We all long for fame and fortune—or at least the fortune part. My husband, a classic introvert and slight misanthrope, would crawl under a rock if fame somehow happened upon him. So he says. It's still hard for me to fully believe; I had Hollywood dreams the second my feet hit the American pavement . . . of the *Jerry Springer* variety.

Consuming copious amounts of *The Oprah Winfrey Show, Sally Jessy Raphaël, Jenny Jones, Ricki Lake*, I dreamed of being a talk show host. "Problems, problems, everyday problems, problems of every-day life," I sang as my intro, forcing my little brother and neighbor onto our white pleather couch.

"Did you cheat on him?" I'd ask the six-year-old neighbor, pointing to Alex or "Tell me how this woman is driving you crazy," I'd instruct him.

When I was in junior high, my parents, likely concerned about my lack of a social outlet, enrolled me in Lee Strasberg Theatre and Film Institute near Union Square. Its red door enclosed yet another world I didn't belong in. Nevertheless, I looked forward to my Satur-day classes where I watched city theater kids cry on cue and emote to an eye-popping degree. And I made the acquaintance of two less than popular girls who I grabbed lunch with at *Subway* during our breaks. One of them was named Scarlett Johansson.

I always thought I was not liked because I was less than—less cool, less confident, less American. Yet, it was obvious that Scarlett was not liked by other budding actresses because she was *more* than. This was my first glimpse at how shining can alienate you as much as wilting—either way, you're an outsider.

Later, I spent years pursuing a hosting and acting career, and while I had some little spotlight moments, they all fell short. Big roles, big money, lots of fame—that's what I yearned for. Until I stopped. Living in Los Angeles amongst thousands of dreamers like myself, I found the part of me that didn't care about worldly success.

I communed with nature, hiking and doing yoga outdoors. I read books. I reached for peace. Ironically, in my tiny room in the princess tower of an old Hollywood building, I let go of my Hollywood dreams.

I went back home to New York, to my family. I met my husband, I gave birth to my daughters.

And then the specter of fantasy crawled back into my psyche. Slowly, I began dreaming once more. This time though, I'm trying to focus on what makes me come alive as well as how I can be useful to others. Over and over, I retrieve my mind from the mirage of glittery outcomes, bringing it back to the present moment.

"I can't help it, I just can't help it," Charlie says when she can't make herself eat a new food or can't stop herself from doing something she knows she shouldn't. I feel the same way: I *want* to break my habit of obsessing about success but, sometimes, I just can't help it. The Tao Te Ching, though, reminds me to try, as well as to change my definition of "success." Because if we limit it to mean riches and accolades, we are setting ourselves up for a rude awakening.

Even if we get there—reach some "out there" achievement—we will still have our inner struggles to deal with. Nothing outside of ourselves can fix us. Just think of how many rich and famous people have ended up in rehab or died by suicide. The Hollywood divorce rate is roughly two times higher than that of the general population. Surely then, fame and fortune do not guarantee happiness.

"But if it were me, I wouldn't fuck it up," many of us think. And maybe we wouldn't. Then again, maybe we would.

Money and power do not change who we are on the inside; they just give us a bigger canvas. If we haven't yet dealt with our baggage, this could mean creating bigger messes.

The Tao instructs us to "have faith in the way things are." Do your work, trust yourself and the Universe, be of service when you can. The rest will take care of itself.

The Trap

You know how when you've got something on your mind, you start seeing it everywhere you go? Synchronicity. We're told, "See the world as yourself"—a mirror for your psyche, an extension of your soul, and vice versa—because it is.

As I was pondering our obsession with success, I stumbled upon an episode of Dax Shepard's podcast, *The Armchair Expert*, where he interviewed Professor of Positive Psychology Tal Ben-Shahar. This guy's lectures on happiness were Harvard's most packed lectures ever. In discussing the rise of systemic depression throughout the world, the professor pointed to our society's myth of success as the culprit.

Our problem, he explained, is we are plagued by thinking when we get A or accomplish B, we will be happy. But that's an external view of success and happiness. Even if A or B come to fruition, our conditional happiness is short-lived.

This human tendency is known as the hedonic treadmill—a theory in which we eventually return to status quo despite major positive or negative life changes. For instance, as a person makes a lot of money, expectations and desires increase as well, resulting in no permanent gain in happiness. So, instead, positive psychologists like Ben-Shahar work to uncover ways to make lasting changes to our mood—all of which are internally motivated.

That's what I'm into, I decided: positive psychology with a side of spirit.

Unlike the many years I tried to hide my crazy, I now consider my mental health a full-time job, much like motherhood. Antidepressants are part of the picture, as is regular exercise. In fact, Ben-Shahar says physical activity may accomplish even more for our mental well-being than medications. The form of this physical activity is up to us, of course—a kid-centered living-room dance party counts every bit in my world—so long as it gets those endorphins flowing.

I've also found my mood suffers when I do, do, do endlessly, trying to achieve and check items off my task list. I need to balance movement with nothingness or with inspiration on a daily basis, planting my two feet on the ground through *being* rather than through *doing*. I yearn for at least a modicum of unstructured time with my family (although in quarantine days, I might have gotten more than I bargained for). I benefit from hikes in nature and have a nightly ritual with my cat, petting him on the stoop or watching him frolic as I inhale the evening air.

I choose a thousand big and little things to help me feel good. I hope you do as well. And if you don't, I hope you will.

Do Your Tao

Commit to dismounting the Hedonic Treadmill. Rather than wholly working your butt off towards your goals, give yourself a daily reprieve to just "be." Set limits for the efforts you're applying to future happiness and success and carve out space for simply feeling good *now* (this isn't the same as lounging around watching TV, though God knows, it's my most craved pastime—but this practice goes a little deeper). Perhaps, allot some time for a nature walk or a book you've been meaning to read. Make a list of all of the things you'd like to start doing more regularly: taking a long bath, stretching, doing a craft with your child, breathing more deeply—and start doing them. During quarantine, those were the very activities that kept me and many others lucid.

Do nothingness works! With simple, daily breaks, we greatly improve our quality of life. Of course, there are periods that are busier than others, but any length of time we can afford will do—even fifteen minutes of stillness can save our sanity.

39

It's All Good

Stop thinking, and end your problems.
What difference between yes and no?
What difference between success and failure?
Must you value what others value, avoid what others avoid?
How ridiculous!
This takes one far from the ultimate Truth.

The crowds are busy with their routines as if they were attending a feast.
I alone am unconcerned—the future seems unknown just like an
*   infant's future.*

They appear to have more than enough;
I alone seem to possess nothing.
I am but a guest in this world, like someone without a home.

Other people have purpose;
I alone don't know.
I seem to drift on a directionless journey like a wave on the ocean,
I blow as aimless as the wind.

Indeed I am different . . .
I have no treasure but the Eternal Mother,
I have no food but what comes from her breast.

—TAO TE CHING, VERSE 20

So, here's our new motto:

It's. All. Good.

I Am But a Vagabond

I am a vagabond. At heart, anyway, I am a drifter—though I prefer "dreamer." These days, I live in a lovely home. I have a husband, two kids, a station wagon, and a will. People even call me "ma'am." I pack lunches and sign permission slips. But at heart, I am still an immigrant kid finding my way. And I'm a dreamer.

I can tell you this now with neither pride nor shame—it's simply a fact—though in my earlier adulthood, it was a source of embarrassment and of suffering. Needlessly, I thought something was wrong with me; I felt like a loser, like a failure to launch. Yet this verse of the Tao Te Ching tells me it's okay to embrace myself—who I've been and who I still am, beneath the surface.

If you feel directionless, if you feel "as aimless as the wind," I invite you to embrace it as well! Don't try to tether yourself.

When I first moved to America, I did all I could to fit in. Somewhere along the way, I lost my footing. By college, I became depressed, lost. And after college, as my friends established their identities in nine-to-five—or nine-to-as-late-as-needed—jobs, I stalled, searched, and slept. I slept a lot. I slept so much some days, it felt as if I were catching up on all my future sleep deprivation.

I took a TV journalism course; I got a job as a news writer, then a news reporter. Yet, something still didn't sit right within me. I wanted the destination but couldn't figure out the journey.

I traveled to Chicago for a hosting opportunity. I got some on-air work interviewing businessmen at the American Stock Exchange. But in between these seemingly cool occasional gigs, I had way more downtime than money in my pocket. In hindsight, it was in those empty stretches that I found myself—I read endless books, I studied yoga and Reiki, I searched for meaning. Back then though, still living with my parents, I hid away from the world in angst, ashamed of my inadequacies.

By the time I met Adam, I'd established only a modicum of normalcy. I had a low-paying job; I rented a cheap room from my friends, part of which was curtained off to store their stuff—his golf clubs, her violin. (I've accumulated *stuff* now too; back then I lived light.)

When we decided I would officially move into Adam's apartment, I brought over the remainder of my things in several plastic bags and on a bunch of hangers. I say "remainder" because I'd filled up a drawer by then, along with some closet space—which is all I really needed.

"Where's the rest of your stuff?" he asked looking at my haphazard armful.

"This is it," I said.

I think the minimalist part of him was impressed, while the worldly part was freaked out.

"I'm just a vagabond," I shrugged and we went on with our lives.

Yes, No . . . Whatever

If you are reading this, it means I've made it. It means I've done something rather decent with myself, with my abilities. I wrote something that actually got published. I am an author. I will say it again just for fun: I. Am. An. Author. But as much as I want to celebrate this and rejoice, I know I must give credence to every failure I've ever experienced. Because I want you to know what I wish someone had told me—no matter where you are on the success metric, it's all good!

I cannot put a number on how many times I have failed. Hundreds, I would have to guess. While my successes I can count on one hand, maybe two if I'm being kind to myself. But this makes sense: it's our falls, our shortcomings that shape us and clear the field for the eventual triumphs. Really, when we're celebrating our accomplishments, we are celebrating every blunder, every defeat, every bout of idleness that came beforehand—because where we are is a summation of where we've been and what we've learned.

"What difference between yes and no? What difference between success and failure?" Lao Tzu asks us. Until we learn to be at peace with the noes, the yeses can be slow to come.

I remember trying so hard to get pregnant with Charlie. It was awkward, frustrating, and the opposite of sexy, as Adam would tell you. I realized I had to let go of my efforts—and then she came. I am in no way trivializing the problem of infertility, which is so real and so painful for many couples. But I know of those who stopped *trying* to get pregnant, stopped the endless IVF, and then miraculously conceived on their own. Or eventually the treatments worked and they had an even greater appreciation of their little souls than the rest of us. And I know parents who went through hell for years and then decided to adopt, now embodying a blissful family. There are also couples who couldn't have a child and made peace with that, finding fulfillment through other avenues, succeeding elsewhere.

"Bring acceptance into your non-acceptance," wrote Eckhart Tolle in *The Power of Now*, "Bring surrender into your non-surrender. Then see what happens."

When I did in fact get pregnant, I really, honestly thought I would be satisfied forevermore. But, of course, we are not built that way, are we? Before long, I wanted another baby. And after that baby, I returned to the struggle that's always haunted me—the quest for some sort of accomplishment, for a more solid presence.

I know now, that even when what we want arrives, we'll want for something else, then something else, and so forth—such is our human nature. I am learning to identify, at least a part of the time, with the higher Me—the one that doesn't care either way, but is serene. The one that's happy to blow with the wind.

Do Your Tao

I dare you, in this moment, to release your greatest dream to the Universe. Say it out loud or write it down or both—and keep it in the present.

Me: "I'm a bestselling author, dammit . . . this book gets around like wildfire." That's all I got for now. I close my eyes and let the Universe talk back.

Universe: [Crickets.] Seriously: crickets outside my window.

Me (in my head): "But what if . . ." "and nothing happens . . ." "and bad, bad, blah, blah, blah." I shut my eyes tighter and breathe. I feel the pulse of the world—no, of the Universe. I trust the pulse. I know it will take care of me. All is well.

Now you!

40

Captain of My Fridge

She who understands others is wise;
she who understands herself is wiser.
She who conquers others is strong;
she who conquers herself has true power.

If you know you have enough, you are truly rich.
If you stay in the center and embrace death, you will endure forever.

—TAO TE CHING, VERSE 33

Or

When you learn to master yourself—your thoughts, your habits,
your compulsions—
the whole world is your freakin' oyster.

Self-Mastery

The reason I am so profoundly grateful for all of my problems and inadequacies is because to get over them, I needed to master myself. And as the Tao Te Ching implies, this is the greatest of powers.

"What doesn't kill you makes you stronger," in other words.

I actually chose that quote for my high school yearbook, right under my very-serious-trying-to-look-sexy photograph. I was far from healthy then—entangled in a codependent teenage relationship, smoking, doing drugs (not the good kind), having never dealt with my secret tween eating disorder, it lay dormant at the time, only to come back to haunt me after my hot-and-heavy eighteen-year-old love affair shattered.

But this quotation, attributed to German philosopher Friedrich Nietzsche turned out to be true, prophetic almost. When I picked the austere words, I had been referring to my common, laughable teen dramas: a best friend who'd stolen my boyfriend, the feeling that I didn't belong. My true strength came later, in my eventual— perhaps, delayed—adulthood.

I'd felt a lack of control for many years and subconsciously drowned in victimhood—born poor in a "bad" country, shuffled from one place to another as a child, bullied, then overlooked, then objectified. I had turned all of these external circumstances upon myself, attacking my body as the host of a suffering soul. First I starved myself; then, when I could no longer stay away from food, with its scents and textures and life, I became bulimic. Cue the damned violins; endless misery ensued . . . well, not endless.

I clearly remember the moment of reckoning when I knew it was *I* who needed to change, I who had the power to alter my existence. Having yet again expunged an enormous amount of food, I knelt on the bathroom floor feeling weak, so sad, beyond saving. Though I seemed to have flushed my self-hatred down the toilet, it still felt like it would swallow me whole. *A waste of human space,* I thought, *disgusting, living for nothing.*

And yet, in the deepest abyss of hopelessness, I heard or felt or sensed a strong presence—an energy far greater than my worldly problems. Now I would refer to it as the Tao or Spirit. Then, I saw it as an awakening—my first experience of becoming the observer of my own human turmoil, seeing it for what it was: a blip in time, a bottom from which I was yet to rise. So, eventually that is what I did.

I committed to my mental health, I sought psychotherapy and loads of therapeutic books. My progress was intermittent; there were times I fell off the wagon—like when my first therapist placed a giant cookie tray in front of me and proceeded to fall asleep in the middle of our session. Still, my addiction to using food as comfort lessened over time. At first, I stayed away from indulgent trigger fare like pizza, fries, donuts—but, one day, I turned around and realized I was free. Gradually, then all of a sudden, food lost its control over me and the strength within me was all that mattered.

Nowadays, I mostly eat to live, not the other way around. I mean, I take pleasure in nightly or daily treats, or both. But it's really more of a mental state: a chance to relax and indulge, or to enjoy the ambience of an intimate meal out. This doesn't mean I don't stuff my face occasionally—I do, though even then, I choose to not give a flying fuck. I think a part of me is actually proud of how little I care now. Food itself is not something I think about, other than in a utilitarian manner, as in feeding the family or appeasing my own physical hunger. I've divested it of its negative power. In fact, my addictive personality, which was also behind my obsessive behavior with men, is mostly tamed. It still rears its persistent head, sure—these days in the form of uncontrollable scrolling or a hankering for some sort of buzz—but I intend daily to fill that void with a connection to the mystical, the Tao, the pure love I feel for my babies (especially when they're asleep!), or with trees and sunsets and rivers and so on. Or, I don't fill the void and smoke it instead . . . whatever. At least somewhere within me, I understand that the choice is mine.

My freedom comes from self-mastery, a lifetime of mishaps behind it. I am a small but mighty, human yet all-powerful. As William Ernest Henley wrote in the poem "Invictus," "I am the master of my fate, I am the captain of my soul"—or at least my fridge.

And so are you.

Do Your Tao

What part of yourself have you yet to master? I, along with the Tao Te Ching, want to encourage you to do it.

The key to self-mastery is a decision—an agreement you make and often remake with yourself, followed by patience, forgiveness, and a million teeny-tiny steps. In Alcoholics Anonymous, their motto is "Just for today." One day at a time. It's the same motto that got us through the rough patches of quarantine.

Self-mastery, though, is a lifelong process, and it's not always about overcoming a detrimental behavior or situation. It can be a commitment to writing regularly, for instance, like I made with myself a couple years ago. I have a friend who, as an adult, committed to playing the piano daily and painting weekly. For some, mastering themselves means weight loss and for others, it's learning to love their body.

My current self-mastery project is to let go of future outcomes, to relish joyful moments, to *be* in the moment (you know, the usual gobbledygook that is my bread and butter).

Whatever it is that you want or need to do, you can do it. Make the decision and then take regular small, perhaps, infinitesimal steps towards your vision.

41

Lean Out

The Tao is eternal, the Earth is long-enduring.
Why is this so?
They do not live for themselves,
thus they are present for all beings.

The Master stays behind, that is why she is ahead.
She detaches herself from all things, that is why she is one with them.
By letting go of the self, she is perfectly fulfilled.

—Tao Te Ching, Verse 7

For us mere earthlings,

Get reacquainted with the greater You, the godly observer that
sees beauty everywhere.
Let that capital You take charge once in a while—
giving of yourself, celebrating the success of others, and marveling
at life's bounty.

Filling Up

Fulfillment—that which we are told the Master has achieved—is what we all inherently search for. We may not know how to explain it; we often refer to it as happiness, but that's not quite it, is it? *Full*-fillment, that feeling of being satiated, is both hard and easy to attain, because our truest fulfillment is dependent on nothing more than our very existence. On the other hand, this pure understanding takes mindfulness—sometimes it even looks like complete detachment. As I explained in chapter 4, the act of disappearing was a holy experience for me, my identity gone in service of my baby. However, it is not a state I can exist in for the rest of my life (no one really can).

So how do we find fulfillment in our daily lives, which are crammed with our neuroses, entanglements, busywork, and which we view from our limited vantage point? How do we see beyond it without losing ourselves completely?

I believe detachment needs to be balanced with its opposite: the full expression of your truest self. These seemingly polar experiences— leaving yourself and becoming fully yourself—bring you to the same place: the greater You that is at one with everything else. The goal is to connect and reconnect, time and time again, with this capital You beyond the you—this part of yourself that is more than just your earthly desires and that stems directly from the Tao, the Universe, God. This You is infinite and extends much further than your physical form. When you align yourself with it, you tap into endless possibility.

Paradoxically, as you surpass your worldly needs, you are actually able to attain them. The Tao may be far grander than our human goals and desires but it also makes them easier to reach—it is "present for all beings." In realizing you are one with it, you cease to struggle. You open up like a flower, receiving the gifts of the Universe. Love then pours out of you more naturally than ever. Your generosity becomes automatic, like that of nature itself—the giving and taking turns into an organic dance.

Falling Behind

Take a look at how people act on the road, behind their steering wheels, and you get a good snapshot of where we are as a society. For some, it seems as if all their anger is channeled into those honks of the horn and lewd gestures; they will crash their own car before they let you through. On the other hand, you witness folks who gracefully usher you in, blinking their blinkers in quick succession to let you know you can go, you are welcome.

Of course, I aim to be like the latter group, on the road and in my life. This necessitates a constant reminder to self: don't honk, let him through, give love freely, don't worry about being usurped, share your secrets.

In the only serious writing class I ever took—a cornucopia of adults with outlandish, heart-breaking, inspiring stories—my teacher would encourage us to be good literary citizens: praise others, write positive reviews, share tips, buy books. This principle can be applied to any area you'd like to succeed in. Want to get ahead? Help others on their journey. Want to make money? Tip large. Want to find love? Be genuinely happy for those who have. And remember to extend this generosity to your imperfect self.

Because we are human, we have off days when our ego gets the best of us; we can be petty, obsessive, belligerent. I used to tear myself apart after such episodes. I felt like a fraud.

But when Charlie once witnessed me lose control, she came up with the perfect explanation. "I know what you have, mommy," she told me as I sat there sulking. "You have the terrible twos."

The "terrible twos," the "threenager threes"—we've found all sorts of monikers for the tantrums thrown by our children, whose brains are simply not developed enough to handle big emotions. Well, sometimes our brains or our spirits aren't either.

Ah, those terrible thirty-nines again, I now think when my impatience, frustration, anxiety gets the better of me, and I let it go.

Forgive yourself when you screw up. Remedy what you can and simply let yourself fall behind when you feel like it. Whether you've hit pause on your spiritual journey or your ambitions, be okay with it. You're allowed to take your time—life is not a race. Or as one Russian proverb puts it, "the slower you go, the farther you'll get."

Funny enough, a big-time agent quoted this to me when I told him where I was born. We had a long, full conversation; then he ghosted me. The quote remained.

Do Your Tao

Ride the wave of the Tao and remember to be grateful for everything you have, starting with life itself. If you can cultivate internal happiness, you are ahead of all the strivers. Whatever else comes along, your cup runneth over!

I'm sure you've heard of a gratitude journal, which I know I've tried and dropped and tried again. Perhaps it's time to start our own version of one, even if it's only in our heads. Try this for the next few nights: as you get into bed, make a list (mental or on paper) of everything that fulfills you—as in fills you up. On bleak days look for the smallest things that have gone right, like having a satiating meal, a conversation, a welcoming pillow, or a laugh—even if merely TV-induced. Get into the habit of balancing your desires with acknowledgment of what fills you up from the inside out—on the most physiological level, the blood flowing through your veins, the neurons firing in your brain . . . and don't forget the thoughts, which you can direct to fulfill you even more:

"I am alive."

"I've come so far."

And as God said to Moses in the Old Testament, "I am that I am."

42

Do Not Force

Those who lead by following the Tao do not use force to conquer
the world.
For every force there is a counterforce.

The Master does his job and then stops.
He understands that the Universe is forever out of control,
and that trying to dominate events goes against the current of
the Tao.
Because he believes in himself, he doesn't try to convince others.
Because he is content with himself, he doesn't need others' approval.
Because he accepts himself, the whole world accepts him.

Remember that good results follow natural law.
They are not brought about by forcing the course of events.

—TAO TE CHING, VERSE 30

So,

Stop trying to hammer what you want into being!

A Forced Career

I've read this verse countless times, and yet, its sentiment cannot be repeated often enough. Do Not Force. *Do Not Force*, I want to yell at myself and everyone who will listen. Holding myself back doesn't come naturally to me. Born a rather type-A personality in the most rigid of societies, I want to hammer my desires into being. I want to push until I get what I want. Of course, this type of manic effort hasn't gotten me anywhere. Trying to force love always landed me alone and in tears. And whenever I battled for my dazzling dreams, I was left confused, bereft of clarity.

I still feel a hot sense of shame when I remember emailing producer after producer at Nickelodeon and the Disney Channel, sending them videos of my reporting, proclaiming my (true) love of kids. I'm not sure what I thought I'd accomplish—I just wanted a chance—perhaps an audition for *Blue's Clues*? At one point, one of the "important" folks I'd reached out to called me up to yell at me.

"Stop harassing all these busy people," he told me. "Get an agent," and he hung up. My force, my belief that I could beat my future into existence backfired in a shame spiral.

Even today, as a writer, I must hold myself back from endlessly contacting editors. There's still a part of my brain that thinks if I push hard enough, I can push my way through. I recently edited an essay into what I thought was a better, more timely version and sent it to someone who had already rejected the original. She seemed pissed off when she told me as much. My one-track mind got me in trouble yet again, and for a second, I was once more that naïve kid getting yelled at by someone "important."

A Watched Pot

While ease versus force may be a never-ending assignment for me, thankfully, life—mostly in the form of children—necessitates that I put my bottomless ambitions on the back burner. And that's when things seem to work out, as if all on their own.

When I submitted a piece of writing to the *New York Times* in my dozenth attempt, I actually managed to forget about it—an unusual occurrence. Summer vacation had just begun for my kids, and so each day, my goal was to entertain and to survive.

As I took my older daughter to her very first movie, I nonchalantly checked my phone during previews. With *Toy Story 4* about to begin, I learned I was to get my biggest writing break to date. Reading the *New York Times* editor's email informing me they will be using my story, I had to think back to remember which one she was talking about. The piece in question had been born out of a love for my children—a singular moment of mayhem that spawned my musings on raising first-generation Americans. In a beautiful, Tao-orchestrated circle, I forgot about my pursuit while taking care of said children and discovered its success during a special moment with my girl.

I've been chasing this state of forgetfulness ever since—but of course, whatever we chase is elusive. Regardless, I recognize that my dreams actualize in the absence of pushing or in a state of alignment. And I suspect the secret to true success is not killing yourself to get what you want, but rather adopting an air of *I don't give a fuck.*

So, go after your dreams but then let go. As many spiritual teachings tell us, tying your happiness to success may actually preclude you from succeeding.

Pushback

It's fascinating to me that long before Isaac Newton came along, Lao Tzu summed up one of his most famous findings—Newton's Third Law of Motion: For every action, there is an equal and opposite reaction. "For every force, there is a counterforce."

Just as I was contemplating this truth, a young woman texted me asking for advice on her relationship. She was annoyed with her boyfriend for something she perceived he was lacking and wanted to know how she should communicate this issue. The truth is, I didn't really have an answer. All I knew is that trying to change another person is a fruitless endeavor. More so, it has negative consequences; such is the law. I told her as much. I said to talk to him about it only if she could do so without blame and definitely without force—something I don't always adhere to myself. It's easier to give advice than to live it, right?

The fact is, when you pressure another person, in one form or another, they will push back. Every parent has experienced admonishing a little kid only to have them perpetuate the behavior in question even more. And many of us have learned the hard way that pressuring for commitment only makes our object of affection yearn to be set free.

In all relationships, we need to remember that the essence of happiness is freedom. Try to impede another's liberty and they will react adversely. This is true in every arena, in family life as much as in the outside world. So let's take force and the air of desperation out of all our pursuits!

Do Your Tao

What are you pursuing at the moment?

I know when I want something intensely, I can taste it, see it, feel it. And I also fear that it won't happen. If I were to act from a place of fear, I would surely try to force things, but I know my fear would push back—sometimes in the form of a mean executive. I am not interested in that tug of war anymore: fear/force, force/fear, and so on. Instead, I opt to practice a bit of *I don't give a bleep*-ness, along with the manifestation processes in the following chapters—back and forth I go, from creating to allowing, from allowing to creating.

So, whatever it is that you're after—even if it's simply figuring out what that is—try giving your quest some space. You can visualize it floating amidst the clouds, surrounded by that very space. You don't have to know how you'll get there or even *if* you'll get there. Just enjoy it up there in the sky, light and airy. Tell yourself, "I'm breezy." And be breezy.

· ·

go after your dreams
but then let go

· ·

43

ManifesTao'tion

Which means more to you, you or your renown?
Money or happiness: which is more valuable?
I say, what you gain is more trouble than what you lose.

Greater cost comes with greater craving,
greater loss comes from calculating the biggest gains.

Be content; rest in your own fullness.
When you realize there is nothing lacking, the whole world belongs
*   to you.*

—TAO TE CHING, VERSE 44

Get it?

You can only have what you desire when you realize it's not
lacking.

Dissatisfaction

Despite knowing better, there are times when dissatisfaction bubbles within me like carbonated water. I have everything, I know that. I should be grateful, yes. But when I "should" on myself, it only makes me more dissatisfied. And so I yearn ferverntly in those moments—I vie to be seen and to be heard—I covet the very "renown" Lao Tzu spoke of.

I used to beat myself up for this not-quite-eradicated longing, until I understood that it's part of our complex human condition. My husband craves more adventure; my friend, more money; older moms yearn for more attention from their grown children; and on and on and on.

This wanting of ours is natural; at times, it is necessary. Every immigrant like myself emerged from the longing for more; each one of us is a carrier of one hell of a dream, or at least, the child of such carriers. We had to leave the known behind for a shot, a chance at something better, yet as the wanters, we rescind all status. Often seen as less than, we immigrants are actually the carriers of light and of dreams.

Thanks to my parents' vision of a better life, Alex and I got to grow up in a nation full of potholes and possibilities that are ours to navigate. The only problem is—especially in this country of consumption—where does our immense longing end?

Whole industries were built upon our human insecurities: advertising that taps into our ever-growing needs, the fashion mags that pedaled the unattainable beauty I blindly strove for, social platforms, and, yes, even self-help. That is why the Tao Te Ching's reminder is so relevant. Amidst the healthy goals that lead us to build better lives, we must learn to pause and to take stock of all we've got. Because often nothing is actually missing.

You can move towards the future from a place of desperation or from a place of contentment. I don't need to tell you which is more effective. Not to mention that living from contentment is way more enjoyable.

Manifestation

In recent months, I've finally understood that we <u>cannot</u> have what we are wanting.

Do you get it?

If you are desperate to have something, it *cannot* be yours. Think about it energetically. The energy of badly wanting something and the energy of having it are in very different planes. That is why, often, people are only able to get what they yearn for once they release it. We are creative beings—literally—we create the world around us with our thoughts, our actions, our energy. When we beg the Universe for something over and over again, we are stuck in the not-having of it. The Tao says in realizing there is nothing lacking, the whole world belongs to us. If we dwell in lack, it can't. When we dwell in contentment, it does!

This works in ways large and small (of course there isn't small or large for the Universe—just *is*-ness). As you learn to recognize manifestations, you see them in your everyday life, which then transforms from ordinary to extraordinary. This happened to me many months into the pandemic, when after a quick, masked trip to Starbucks with my kids, I was sad. It felt like our society had forgotten how to connect—nobody even gazed in our direction, including while Gigi performed a loud, stompy dance in between all the roped-off tables. Everyone seemed so separate from one another and I longed for the days of old. As 2021 rolled around, I wrote about this experience and about my wish for a re-emergence of humanness. I expressed my hopes of feeling connected to strangers once more; I reveled in the thought of mundane smiles and conversations. And then I moved on. Just envisioning a friendlier future made me happy.

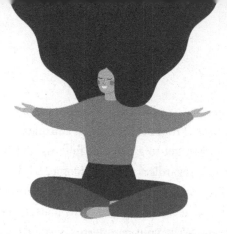

The next time Gigi and I went to that very same Starbucks, a barista immediately handed her a free cake pop—"Sometimes you just gotta spread kindness," he said. Another customer struck up a conversation with us; everyone seemed to smile, even through masks. It was as if the world had been transformed. I remembered that when we change our outlook, we do change the world—we shift the entire Universe. But that can only occur when we let go of the reins; we cannot push or plead it into existence.

Want more proof of our ability to manifest once we relax and "rest in [our] own fullness"?

You. You are the proof.

The fact that you're taking in my words this very instant is proof that we can manifest our dreams once we learn how to be content regardless, because you, my friend, are helping carry out my dream. And I totally get how New Agey this sounds—vision boards, life maps, *The Secret*—even the New Age stuff feels stale. Still, if you envision, hope, and, most importantly, *believe* that a certain reality can be yours . . . well, you have a much better chance than begging for it.

Sometimes it is all BS. But sometimes it is not. That is totally up to you. If you do all the "right" activities in an effort to manifest your desires, but inside you feel manic and desperate, they are for naught. It is better to stop and simply realize there is nothing lacking.

Do Your Tao

If you are desperate to succeed, you cannot succeed, no matter how hard you push. From networking to affirmation cards—it's all swell, *if* it helps you get to a place of fullness and hopefulness—pre-manifestation, regardless of the outcome. So do whatever you can to be fulfilled *now* and release your expectations. When you get to that feeling place, nothing else really matters. Feel good, feel glad, feel at peace. Write your manifestos, visualize your zen-ness, take your actions from there.

As the Tao asks us, "Money or happiness: which is more valuable?" I mean, c'mon, is there anything more valuable than happiness?

Get to the happiness first; get there regardless! If you can make your internal experience more significant than external outcomes, you are free. You *are* successful.

44

The Sixth Sense

In order to shrink something, you must first allow it to expand.
In order to weaken something, you must first allow it to strengthen.
In order to get rid of something, you must first allow it to flourish.
In order to possess something, you must first give it away.

This is called subtle understanding:
the soft and pliable overcomes the hard and inflexible.

Just as fish remain hidden in deep waters,
Keep your workings a mystery.

—TAO TE CHING, VERSE 36

Also,

This subtle understanding of everything is available to you, always.
Let yourself be soft, take your time . . . simply perceive it.

Precognition

I once dreamt of writing a book. I had this dream lurking in my sub-
conscious, way before I was writing regularly (and not at all, most of
the time). Still, I told my friend at twenty, or some such very young
big-eyed age, that I think one day I will write a book.

"But a book about what?" she asked.

"Oh, I don't know, about my life, I guess," I answered and
promptly forgot about it.

I forgot long enough to live a life of confusion and endless trial
and error, to love and lose and grasp and fail—basically, I let go of my
out-of-nowhere declaration long enough to be given the materials
for this very tome I was to produce.

This has always been the case with me. Out-of-nowhere declarations that *feel* true.

"I'm worried about dad," I kept annoying my mom. He got very
ill from COVID-19 soon after.

And, "I'll meet someone in time for your wedding," I'd told my
bestie Carolyn, insisting she keep my number at two, a.k.a. *plus one*,
for the event.

"Yikes, that's a lot of pressure," she said, not quite knowing what
to make of my resolve.

The thing is, it wasn't even a goal—not this time, anyway—it
just was. I knew I was ready for "the one," or rather, "*a* one," beyond
logic, beyond doubt. Adam, as you might have guessed, was my date
to the wedding.

I've always known things slightly ahead of time. In some part
of our being, we all do. It's heeding our subtle perception that's the
hard part. This sixth sense is not something we need to learn, but,
rather to remember—an impulse like that of an animal in the wild. I
look my weathered Regis in the eye and know he knows that I know.
What I know is, he's in line with the Tao, with all of existence, and
that a cat's piercing intuitiveness is something we all can access.

Intuition

I stumbled upon the concept of intuition when I was fourteen years old, already confused but not yet despondent. Staying at an aunt's in New Jersey, I asked to go to Barnes & Noble where I beelined for the spiritual section (or was it self-help?). I picked up only one book, as if completing an errand—though I hadn't had a plan in mind whatsoever—and headed for the register. The book was titled *Practical Intuition*.

Author Laura Day's words reminded me—at that tender age—of an ability I wasn't even sure I had. Dutifully doing the exercises outlined by this renowned psychic (she prefers the term "intuitive"), I got in touch with my own psychic powers, which Laura swears everyone possesses. She was almost a mythical figure to me—this small, stylish woman I had seen on *The Oprah Winfrey Show*, whose harrowing childhood made her rely on intuition more than most of us. *I can foresee things too*, I realized, and then once again forgot all about it, misplacing her book somewhere in the depths of my teenage drama.

Years later, with my life at a standstill, I was back at Barnes & Noble, finding comfort amongst its aisles, its sameness. I came to catch Laura Day's free one-hour presentation. More than a decade after magically plucking her work out of a sea of books, I sat listening to her speak. She became an important part of my life—I joined a group of women who workshopped her books—part of a fluid community she calls "The Circle." A struggling actress, as I thought of myself, I was permitted to attend her weekend intensive merely by helping to stack some chairs. And then once more in 2020, with the world in a tailspin of confusion, I joined this bewitching woman—literally: she's finally acquired a cauldron—in many of her free workshops online.

Ms. Day's generosity has taught me that when you have faith, you give, knowing the stream of goodness that supplies all will not run out on you. She also showed me we can be as powerful and as skillful as we choose—that intuition, like any other ability, is a craft you practice in order to improve it. Most importantly, Laura taught me that I can rely on myself, on my own inner voice to guide the way. When I plug into what I refer to as the Tao or Source—what Laura calls the "Unified Field"—I am able to focus my energy to support my dreams.

Subtle Understanding

Laura Day's work is a source of comfort for homebodies like me—the kind we all became in 2020. I used to feel lazy because of my inability to constantly be moving and shaking like others I'd witnessed. But her teachings helped me feel comfortable with who I was, ensuring I could be masterful even in stillness. In getting comfortable with my "laziness," I became the most sincere, hardworking version of myself. I'm now learning to flow from one state to another as needed, because . . . you can't be lazy when you want to pen a book, right? But what about the part of me that wants to Netflix into oblivion?

Intuition helps me integrate all my parts in order to achieve what I want to achieve, not to mention that wholeness feels so much better than fighting with yourself. When you are aware of what's going on inside you and you align your energy into a singular beam of light—well, your life unfolds with inevitability. So, let's get started!

Do Your Tao

Here's the directive that is the basis of Laura Day's book *The Circle*, which takes us on a journey of creation:

Make a wish. Simple. Go ahead, do it; I mean take all the time you need, but then do it. Make. A. Wish. And, don't worry, if you don't have a clear vision for yourself—your wish can simply be for more clarity (which we can all use).

Now dwell in your wish as if it has already actualized. What does it look like? Experience it as a wish come true with all of your senses. Write down what this practice feels like. In doing so, you may get insights into what needs to change within yourself and in your external life to make room for this dream. Because things don't just come into our lives on top of what already exists there—we must reconfigure bits and pieces of ourselves and our worlds so that the whole picture is more satisfying. But we can lean on intuition to guide us in the right direction.

Start keeping tabs on coincidences—or what we, the spiritual, call synchronicities—as they occur in your daily existence. Where are they leading you? What does your gut want you to do? Don't hurry. Collect the information your intuition is noticing and your wish, your vision, your life will gain more fullness and color.

. . . .

make a wish . . .
dwell in your wish

. . . .

45

Fake It

A great scholar hearing of the Tao, works diligently to embody it.
A middling scholar hearing of the Tao, half believes it, half doubts it.
An inferior scholar hearing of the Tao, laughs and jeers at it.
If he didn't laugh and jeer, it wouldn't be the Tao.

Thus it is said:
the way of the light seems dark,
the way forward seems like retreat,
the sure way seems unsteady.
True power seems weak,
true steadfastness seems changeable,
true clarity seems obscure.
The greatest art seems unsophisticated,
the greatest love seems indifferent,
the greatest wisdom seems childish.

The Tao is hidden and nameless,
yet it nourishes and completes all things.

—Tao Te Ching, Verse 41

So, practically speaking,

Move forward by going back to the origin.
You are God in human form, the Tao in motion—embody that!

20/20 Vision

The Tao reminds us to open up our eyes and look deeper than the surface reality we are presented. "The way of the light seems dark" because the darkness is necessary for the light to emerge brighter. Because beneath every disappointment lies the seed of something greater, in every weakness, a hidden strength, with every tyrant, a call for love. Such is this world of duality. Without its opposite, a thing or state cannot exist, teaches Neale Donald Walsch, the author of *Conversations with God.* And contrast—the bad, the unwanted—provides context. It makes more clear to us what we do want, what we do believe.

It is no surprise, then, that by the end of 2020, everyone was eager to see it go. We seemed to act as if all the world's problems would be carried off with that year—as if it were the enemy, the monster that we were about to slay, bury, and wash our hands of. Of course it was not. It wasn't anything, really . . . merely a label we put on a construct we ourselves had created: the measure of time. Why was it so important then for us to cross it off the calendar?

The yearning for a new beginning was stronger than ever. You could smell it in the air, even with a cloaked nose. But, guess what? You can have this new beginning any time you choose.

Child's Play

What I envision for you and for me—whether at the start of a new year or at any point when we decide to begin anew—is the kind of clarity that spans beyond our external lives and occurrences, beyond what's on the news and on our streaming devices (though I love binge-watching shows as much as the next gal—but you know that already). I hope each of us searchers will come to believe a little more deeply in our potential and in our ability to create ourselves at any time. I hope we connect to the hidden Tao which nourishes all things. Many of us who are into the mystical side of life have glimpsed what this connection with the Universe, the Tao, Source feels like. But once we start seeking it out on a regular basis, we can become the Masters of our own existence.

While the timeless You is eternal, you may not have yet reaped the power of this You in your current physical form. Want to become the kind of person who has?

In order to create something new, something better than what we've created in the past, we must become someone new. Laura Day calls this practice embodiment—the act of embodying a New You— the you that already has whatever it is that you want. For instance, the New Me is confident in her purpose, relaxed in her relationship with others, and is able to quiet her ego in order to operate as her Higher Self. And she has a book out; (duh) you're reading it. I've been working on this New Me for a long time, sometimes consciously, methodically, other times, blindly, clumsily, painfully. Still, this work-in-progress-me is awesome and capable. I am able to embody her much more than I used to. And now, when I slip backward into the old, judgy, lonely, craggy me, the New Me pulls me out rather quickly and easily.

· ·

in order to create something new, we must become someone new

· ·

This embodiment is actually the simplest thing in the world— imagine how, who, where you want to be and pretend to be that person as often as you can remember. It's child's play, really—as the Tao Te Ching says, the greatest wisdom seems childish. This process of embodiment is fun and can feel so good (though silly at first). It can also be uncomfortable. Still, do what kids do—commit to your imagination, go with it. When you pretend to be whoever you want to become, you adopt that New You's way of being. The lines blur and you are able to morph into the future.

And don't be fooled—this play takes courage!

Do Your Tao

Whenever you happen to read this, now is your chance for a *New You* resolution, rather than a New Year's one; time isn't neat and linear anyway like we pretend. Write down or simply conjure in your mind's eye what the ideal you looks like, feels like, lives like. Commit to embodying this New You daily, even if for a short time period. When you find yourself sliding back into your old ways, shapeshift into the preferred version of yourself. It may take countless repetitions, but fake it till you make it, as they say.

If you want to, you can alchemize—this is fact.

So adopt the qualities that an actualized You would have. How does she talk, walk, relate to others? The shifts you make may be imperceptible to an onlooker, but by embodying who you want to be, you'll get to where you want to go. As my friend, the author and activist Jen Pastiloff says, "May I have the courage to be who I say I am."

Little by little, the courage will come.

46

Journeying

What is rooted is easy to nourish, what is not yet manifest is easy to avoid.
What is brittle is easy to break, what is small is easy to scatter.
Prevent problems before they emerge.
Put things in order before they get out of hand.

Remember: a tree that is big enough for you to embrace grew out of a tiny seed.
A journey of a thousand miles begins with a single step.

People often fail in their tasks just as they're about to accomplish them.
So give as much care at the end as in the beginning, then there will be no failure.

The Master takes action by letting things take their course.
He simply reminds people of who they have always been,
and this he does without a stir.

—Tao Te Ching, Verse 64

And here's a Russian addition:

While the eyes fear, the hands do.

Start

"The journey of a thousand miles begins with a single step."

Most of us have heard this more than once, but knew little of the phrase's own journey—that it hailed back thousands of years to the Tao Te Ching, to The Book of the Way—a tome which aimed to explain the grandest and the smallest principles of being human. Yet, with all the analysis and all the interpretation to which the Tao leaves itself open, this wee phrase is as simple as it gets. It is merely inviting us to begin—to just get on the mat, as they say in yoga—to make that first, single step . . . which, of course, is the hardest step of all.

By observing my own inner rhetoric, I've realized how many excuses the mind will come up with to talk us out of going after our dreams—how many scenarios it creates to show us why we will never get to where we want to go, why it's not worth even starting: "It's all been done before; I have nothing new to offer," "The odds are against me," "It's a bad time," "I'm not qualified enough, educated enough, successful enough, _____ enough." God, there are millions of excuses we thrust upon ourselves to keep us exactly where we are—stagnant in our lackluster existence. And that is okay. It is totally fine. There is no one judging our choices but ourselves (and maybe a few others, but screw them). You can be exactly where you want to be and you can be there as long as you want to. But know that one day you will expand into your glory. Whether this happens while you're here in physical form is up to you.

Finish

For me, the fear of starting is not even about the risk involved—which, too, is valid. It is the overwhelming dread of how much there is to do in order to succeed—the magnitude and pressure of the whole endeavor. But as a funny, little Russian saying goes, "While the eyes fear, the hands do."

Let the eyes be afraid, *whatever*—how could they not be with the mountain of work ahead? And simultaneously allow your hands to do what they're meant to do, then allow things to flow. I mean, you'll forget to sometimes, but after you've bent yourself into a frantic pretzel, you'll remember. Take this very book, for instance: writing it is one thing—though I wasn't even sure I could carry that out all the way—but selling it is a whole other ball game which felt like a big, heavy burden I knew nothing about. And who would even want to work on a book that they couldn't sell, that no one would ever read? Who'd want to commit their energy before knowing that their vision would come to fruition? That's yet another fearsome blob of an unknown steering us away from trying.

The Universe, Tao, God is tricky that way, right? There are no guarantees. We cannot wait for proof in order to believe in our visions. So begin anyway. Plant the seed anyway. Plant a bunch of seeds if it makes you feel better; let them sprout all over the damn place, and then just follow the Way. *Your* tree will blossom, that is for certain, but you must give it a chance. Because our society is so obsessed with instant gratification, you must be watchful not to squash or abandon your seedling too soon. What is meant to be yours need not be forced or rushed.

It's ironic that while we can have such a hard time starting something, we are simultaneously so eager to complete it, to rush it to its finish. That is our human nature, but it is not our Tao nature. Deep down, we know it's all about the journey and not the destination—we say it often enough. And yet, how many times have we lost patience too quickly—quit on projects, on relationships, on ourselves, perhaps just shortly before things would have gotten good? If I, in my limited mind, had my way, this book would not have existed. Maybe I would've been a TV star or I would've written a different book a long time ago; the point is, everything I ever yearned for would have already taken place—*bam*, done, finished.

But then I would not be me—the person becoming ever more honest with myself and with the world, the one now committed to finding and living this truth until some day I dissolve into it completely.

Whether it's impatience, frustration, or fear of the work ahead— or of failure or success ("Who am I to be brilliant, gorgeous, talented, fabulous?" as Marianne Williamson wrote)—whatever shape this fear takes, remember, you can feel it and move ahead anyway. One step after another, until you turn around and see the winding shape of a beautiful journey, which you finally realize is eternal.

Do Your Tao

You know what's coming, don't you?

The first step—that initial start to whatever you've been putting off or pushing out of your mind. It is time.

Unless it's not.

That's for you to decide. But I hope this thought will help you feel ready-ish: there will never be a better time—the "right" time, and there will never be the perfect circumstance. The time is now, the circumstances are what they are. Just begin. Take a brisk walk, create your dating profile, start researching that trip, write the first (or last) paragraph or the outline or the elevator pitch, or, or, or . . . And if you've already taken the first step, then take the second, the third, the zillionth—sometimes miles into the journey, a step can feel like the first again—don't overthink it, let yourself gain momentum.

And if you do not feel ready-ish to start, then get ready to be ready. Think of, talk about, visualize whatever it is that you hope to do or be or have. Reread the previous chapters. Journal. Then remember who you have always been, and let the action emerge.

Recognize that you are always on a journey . . . so why not choose your own path?

47

Let It Be Easy

Words born of the mind are not true,
true words are not born of the mind.
Wise men don't need to prove their point,
men who need to prove their point aren't wise.

Those who come to know It do not rely on learning.
Those who rely on learning do not come to know It.

The Master does not set out to accumulate fortune or merit,
yet as she serves the people, she becomes richer,
and as she gives to the people, she gets more.

The Tao nourishes by not forcing;
by not dominating, the Master leads.

—Tao Te Ching, Verse 81

And

Let's allow, utilize, enjoy the magnitude of our own power—
it is effing time!

Mastery

When Charlie began losing her baby teeth and permanent ones sprung up, we told her she needed to brush them twice a day now, no longer skipping the mundane habit.

"For the rest of my life?" she sobbed, "Even on my birthday?"

"You can do whatever you want on your birthday," we agreed, giggling at the gravitas of her existential despair.

Soon after, Gigi told me she feels like there's a remote control making her do everything.

Me too sometimes, I thought to myself.

Because that's how life can seem in this physical realm, right? A robotic existence, a flat plane, an endless task list to check off. But like many an optical illusion, this existence is actually what you choose it to be. Robotic or fluid? Flat or round? Boredom or intention? You choose.

You can work on replacing the shoulds and the feeling of being controlled with flow—finding it, cultivating it, peace-ing and ease-ing and joy-ing. Because as long as you're alive, you are never done or complete; you are never *there*, wherever *there* is, so you might as well be easeful and joyful en route. Hear this, please: *You are never done.* Not spiritually and not otherwise. You're like water that becomes vapor that becomes snow that becomes water again, and so on, ever-shifting, ever-evolving. There are no absolute finish lines.

So, let it be easy-ish, friends: *It*—life, existence, being. A little less ego, a lot more Tao, a little less mind, a lot more soul. A little less task-listing and far more unfolding, allowing, being. And just like brushing teeth, this practice is one we return to over and over again. We get knocked out of the stream, back in we go.

The process of releasing the struggle and flowing with the Tao is as easeful as it gets (even when it's less than easeful).

Whatever happens in this world, *Keep calm and Tao on,* so to speak. Let us neither get swept up in the chaos, nor try to dominate events. Let's instead root ourselves deeper still in the benevolent energy of the Universe. Life will take its course, as the hands move along the face of a clock—a new president, a vaccine, a sigh of relief . . . other problems, other losses, other colossal mishaps, both personal and global—but we will remain in the center through the ups and the downs: open, still, connecting the past, present, and future in the single moment of *now.*

At the center of that clock, we can sense things before they happen, and we can experience them long after. Which is why a certain house feels like your first true home, even if it's already sold—only to make its way back to you a year later, now slightly disheveled but still yours. It is why once or twice in a lifetime, when you first hug someone you're shocked to feel forever barreling towards you like a fact. It's why you utter, "We're going to be friends, I can tell," to a girl you just met in one of your many lonely moments. And why you write words that seem like they've already been written and read and rewritten (which they kind of have been because Microsoft Word failed to save them in one of its mysterious glitches, but even that was part of the screwy magic).

At the center, there's nothing left to learn or to attain, only to know and to be. The eternity of mountains is already in your bones. It speaks for itself, just listen. *You are a drop in the bucket of God,* it tells you, *and you are the ocean. You are in everything and everyone, and they are all in you.* In moments large and small we feel this. We run from it sometimes—the magnitude of our own power—but it waits for us patiently. Because it doesn't matter all that much, whether you or I self-actualize. It doesn't even matter if we burn this whole thing to the ground. Tao, the Universe, Source pulses love regardless.

Don't you wanna find out what it feels like, though? To be this Master, this Moses, this Jesus, this Buddha, this Lao Tzu, this Witch, this Sorceress, this Goddess? I do. I want to feel the gifts I have been given fully. I've studied enough, I've learned enough, I've been schooled enough. Now I just want to feel and to *be* fully. I want to God—as in God'ing and Tao'ing—creating and flowing endlessly.

Do Your Tao

What does God'ing even look like to you?

Don't worry if you don't know. I don't quite know yet myself; it's a huge question. But I exist to find out and to create this experience. Sometimes it feels big and important; other times it's just about chilling and being, or acknowledging my mistakes and continuing. I probably won't know for certain until after this lifetime. What I do know is that I am bigger than my human limitations—my crabbiness, angst, judginess, hurt feelings, insecurities, traumas, and all the rest of the shit that makes me lil' ole me: Jessie Kanzer, née Asya Bronfman. I am *so* much more than that, and even more than the humor, joy, friendliness, and warmth that are also a part of my human form. I think the full me *is* that joy, that love, that faith, but on steroids, as is the full You.

That's what it feels like to God fully, I believe: to be, to spread, to create endless love and joy in all its myriad of forms. What am I going to do with this knowledge? How am I going to God? Well, for the next hour I'm gonna take a walk, buy some groceries, breathe a little deeper, glance up at the sky here and there . . . and for now, that will be enough. Being here now is enough.

I invite you to do this with me—to join me in this moment of nowness and to feel its completeness, wherever you are—to inhale, relax, and exhale. Or to create your own version of Tao'ing, and then to do it again and again, moment by moment. And to forget and then remind yourself to come back here to this peace of beingness, like water flowing over boulders . . .

Remember: no matter what is or isn't happening on the outside, you can choose what goes on on the inside. And if you don't like how it feels, you get to choose again, to begin anew, to change your mind.

Brick by brick, we can Tao ourselves into existence. Step by step, we get to walk the Great Way.

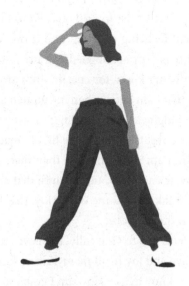

Epilogue

The thing I'd like to tell you here—one last note, if you will, before I shut up for a bit—is that even if you follow none of my suggestions, not a single one, you are doing the Tao. Even if you don't like much of what I've written here, you're doing it and doing it well. Because there is no other way. The "good" and "bad" classifications we give ourselves are simply impositions on *is-ness*, as are all our judgments. Whether I agree with you and like you or not—and vice versa—you and I are one, because that's all there is when we zoom out a bit. And in oneness I extend to you my blessing, my good vibes, my gratitude; I extend it to myself.

Writing this book was an easy feat. It just sorta happened, as if all on its own. It took a span of time, sure, and what we'd call effort (and, oh boy, sleepless nights), but I was able to flow with it then too; I gave myself over to it, not counting the hours and diaper changes it demanded. I know I was but a vehicle here because I asked to be one . . . and now, it's what I yearn for most—more of that connection with Tao, Source, God! That very human *more*.

In this moment, I hope I can gift you what's been gifted to me—though, to mind-bend a little, when it was given to me, it was simultaneously given to you: as I write this, you read this. In the words of Albert Einstein, "The distinction between the past, present and future is only a stubbornly persistent illusion." There are many illusions which make up our agreed-upon reality, including the belief that there is a right way to think, or a right way to be, or a right way to do things. Let yourself dwell in the freedom of knowing there are countless ways to be, do, or have anything.

Find *Your* Way, friend. Tao on!

~JESSIE ASYA KANZER

Acknowledgments

Before I go on thanking all the people in my life there is to thank, I must go to the source: to the Tao itself. As I've said, for me this journey began on the bathroom floor as a mess of a gal. This mess had me searching for anything and everything that could help. When I read James Frey's *A Million Little Pieces*—a book about addiction and recovery—I was touched by the simple, enigmatic words of the Tao Te Ching which he quoted throughout. *The Tao helped him,* I thought, *maybe it will help me.* (James Frey's book then led its own fraught path of criticism and redemption, but for me, it was the start of my Tao'ishness.) I purchased a little pocket edition of Stephen Mitchell's translation of the Tao that has been with me for nearly two decades. Wayne Dyer's *Change Your Thoughts—Change Your Life, Living the Wisdom of the Tao* took me down a rabbit hole that has culminated here, in my own analysis of this text, with my own suggestions for Tao'ing—his thoughtfulness and exercises inspired me greatly, and after he passed I felt compelled to continue this work. Also of great help were Jonathan Star's *The New Translation from Tao Te Ching: The Definitive Edition*, Lok Sang Ho's *The Living Dao: The Art and Way of Living a Rich and Truthful Life*, a translation for public domain by J.H. McDonald, OSHO's *Tao: Its History and Teachings*, and every single person who has ever contributed to spreading the wisdom and simplicity of living the Way.

Susan Shapiro and her NYC writing class were a godsend to me. She helped me see myself as a writer—literally—by helping me get the bylines. I'm so grateful to Beth Wareham for being my guide early on in the process and for bringing me to Lisa Hagan who took me on with gusto—my first agent ever, by the way (in acting I'd only gotten as far as a manager, which somehow was easier to get than an agent, beacause . . . I have no clue . . . humans make things complicated). Lisa brought me to Greg Brandenburgh, whose encouraging, enthusiastic, and just-plain-funny communication kept me afloat through the final stages of this book. Greg's belief in my work solidified my own and I am so thankful to him. And then everyone Greg brought my way at Hampton Roads and Red Wheel/Weiser was supportive and filled me with joy—that there were these helpful people I'd never met shepherding my writing—I could cry. Like my copyeditor Lauren Ayer who I only know through the thorough and motivational notes she left on the side of my pages, and yet we had the intimate relationship of pouring over the same manuscript. My kick-ass, ever-constant supporters: Christine LeBlond, Bonni Hamilton, Eryn Eaton, and the entire Nardi Media team—a big, huge thank you!

It takes a village to birth a book—that is what I've realized through this process—and I appreciate my village very much. You've meant the world to this first-time author.

Thank you to my girlfriends past, present, and future—I am a girls' girl—I revel in your company and complexity, and I root for you; we are one. Thank you to my DF community for your warmth. A huge grazie to Basilio at Café Latte for letting me spend hours there working on this thing and for the complimentary Barolo and the magic environment I needed. And to HudCo, the idyllic space where I first began and then serendipitously edited this book, and to sweet, generous Abbie, who won me a membership there. And to Dear Laura Day and our Circle community for the spiritual support, as well as to my dynamo Elina, for all her priceless advice. And to the village that helps me raise my children, so I can do this, so they

can eventually do some form of this—their teachers, their Ms. Ana
. . . YouTube.

Spasiba to every *Tetya* and *Dyadya* who ever wished me well.
And once again, to my beloved, beloved, beloved girls, my proud
cheerleader family and family-in-law (Hi, Bev!), and to my Adam,
who has made *everything* possible.

About the Author

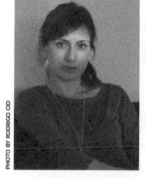

Jessie Asya Kanzer was born in the Soviet Union, and at the age of eight, she emigrated with her family to Brooklyn. She is a writer and former reporter and actress. Her work has appeared in the *Washington Post, New York Daily News, Wall Street Journal, Independent, New York Times, Los Angeles Times,* Huffington Post, Ravishly, and Romper. Jessie lives with her two daughters and husband in Dobbs Ferry, New York. Follow her on Instagram @jessiekanzer

Hampton Roads Publishing Company

. . . for the evolving human spirit

Hampton Roads Publishing Company publishes books on a variety of subjects, including spirituality, health, and other related topics.

For a copy of our latest trade catalog, call (978) 465-0504 or visit our distributor's website at *www.redwheelweiser.com* where you can also sign up for our newsletter and special offers.